Live Long Life

Live Long Life

◆

happy and healthy

Nitin M Patel

iUniverse, Inc.
New York Lincoln Shanghai

Live Long Life
happy and healthy

iUniverse, Inc.

For information address:
iUniverse, Inc.
2021 Pine Lake Road, Suite 100
Lincoln, NE 68512
www.iuniverse.com

ISBN: 0-595-31312-4

Printed in the United States of America

Contents

Preface

Almost all the details discussed in this book have been implemented by me during the long course of time. The book is worth reading and implementing by heart. Do not just read this book, but understand and implement it, and enjoy its unbelievable results on your body, mind and living.

Living up to 100 years is birth the right of every human being. As a matter of fact, God has made our body to last for about 100 years, with the exceptions of some cases of congenital or genetic flaws.

It is up to us how to take care of this wonderful and self-curing body. Taking care of body by good habits and balanced eating, very early in life, is as rewarding as saving money in early life. Early we save, more it will multiply.

Because we can not see the inside of our body, we are not serious enough about the importance of the care and cleaning required for it. We take good care of our house, car, furniture, jewelry, etc., but ignore the important jewel of our life: body and soul.

Read and understand each and every word, sentence, and paragraph. Read again and again to understand its deep meaning. Each paragraph has a link with the following paragraph, and every chapter has a link with the next chapter. So, full attention is required to understand this book in depth.

This book gives details of all aspects of our body, mind and soul, and how they work with one another in harmony, to give us cheerful and happy long life. It may sound difficult to implement it, but with a patient beginning, every step and action will be realized and enjoyed easily and smoothly.

Please have this book in your purse or brief case, inside the drawer of or on your desk or by your bed-side cabinet. Read again and again and understand thoroughly. Start working first on whatever you feel comfortable. Do not just wait to do everything at the same time.

Many great people in India have spent much time of their life to understand the body, mind and soul together. This book is my experiments based on of all such findings of these great people.

I sincerely thank Mr. Arvindbhai P Patel of Vidyanagar, India, for editing this book in a very short time. I also thank Mr. Himanshu Pandya of Shape Communication for his contributions in preparing graphics and cover design.

Hope this book will give what is missing in our modern hectic life.

Nitin Patel
Anand, India
Feb. 12, 2004

1

Life, Living and Longevity

Life:

What is life? The question is simple but the answer requires deep thinking. At one glance, it may look as if life is just time spent between birth and death. Beyond that, we have no idea what the source of our origin was and what our destiny will be.

Who can measure the infinity of time? Life is the interval between birth and death. The journey of the universe is eternal. This is the only life we know, the rest is mystery for eternity. Now it all depends on us as to how and how long to live.

When a human being is born, internal body, with certain exceptions, is clean and able to live for 100 years. After years of living unwisely, we cut short our journey of life. Life is meant for living for a long span. But modern life style has created many diseases, stressful living, tension in society and unhappiness in the end. Due to these artificially created problems, we are not able to live life as it should be.

Life, I mean birth on this wonderful and the only planet where life does exist as human being, is a unique gift of GOD to us. We must appreciate the almighty God that we are born on this planet as healthy and happy human beings. There are about one million specimens on this earth, and human being is the only intelligent and developed creature. We should keep this body as clean and pure as given to us at the time of birth.

Look, for how many years do we live? Say, average 75 or 80 years. Now out of these 75 years, we spend 25 years or, say, one third of our life, in sleeping. Only 50 years are left for living. Again, out of 50 years, we spend a few years in childhood, a few years in preparing for daily routine like bathing, cleaning, etc. So, actually we have been left with only 30 years of our life to live as per our wishes and feelings.

How short the life is! No matter what happen to us, we must enjoy each and every moment with happiness. Life is just limited overs of a game like cricket. Fixed time is given to all of us. It is unfortunate that we cut it short by a wrong style of living, and never play the full game of life.

Living:

"Existence is a fact but living is an art."

Look at the outside world. Birds, animals and many other creatures are living their life. Squandering time is not real living. Real living is where life is full of joy and happiness, and associated with taking and giving, caring and sharing, smiling and calming.

Look at our daily life. Are we living our life? The plain answer is 'no'. We never care about the real happiness of life in the hectic schedule from morning to bed time and after fanciful and trashy ambitions.

Longevity:

To live up to 100 years is our birth right because that is the way God has given us the body and mind at the time of our birth. Look at the children; how innocent and healthy they are! They have no blood pressure, no acidity, no hypertension, and no diabetes. They do not discriminate between different castes, colors, religions, languages or origins. They do not care about anything. They just live their life happy-go-lucky, blithe and breezy. Can we not just make a simple effort to emulate them?

We should live the rest of our life as child. But as we grow up, our mind gets tainted; our health is shattered by wrong eating habits and life style.

Longevity with full joy and happiness can be easily achieved even at any age of life. Just read and understand this book word by word and line by line. Read this book again and again; think deeply over what is written, and then start implementing the suggested steps.

No matter what your age is. If you are serious enough about it, you can bring happiness and joy in your life, with extra years added. It is easy and enjoyable. So start reading this book and get what you should and can get.

2

Body, Breath and Mind

Our body and mind have unique relationship; and both are intimately linked to each other. Whatever happens in the body is a direct reflection of what is going on in the mind. Depression is draining away vitality, while joy is breathing life into the body. Both are strongly bonded and also affect each other. Our existence in this world is spread into these seven layers:

- Body: physical existence
- Breath: felt in and out of body.....
- Mind: boundless power of possibilities
- Intellect: through which this world is developed at this stage
- Memory: witness of happiness and sorrow
- Ego: invisible layer of one's limitations
- Self: soul of body...ultimate reach of divine achievement.

With the combination of Body, Breath and Mind, we can control the rest of our layers of existence. Body is the home of the other six invisible existence of our life. The Intellect, Memory, Ego and Self are controlled by Mind. They are invisible and can only be experienced.

All that we can see is body, but the body is simply a home and nothing else. Therefore, after death, all other six layers of existence stop functioning and the body becomes useless, and finally it is buried or cremated or thrown to birds and animals.

A story of a diamond ring

Let us take an example of a precious diamond ring packed in a nice box. Now, imagine that this is gifted to you. What will you do the next moment? You will put that box in a safe with lock and key, or start wearing that ring immediately. Once you wear that ring, the box will be thrown away, because it has no material value. No matter how nice and good looking that box is, it has no importance to you any more.

Our body and soul has the same relationship. The soul is the diamond ring and the body is the box. But most of the people give more importance to the box (body) and ignore the diamond ring (soul).

The Body:

This body is a complex chemical laboratory and factory. Constant chemical actions and reactions are going on inside the body with the help and command of the mind. The food we eat becomes a chemical compound in a few minutes. After that, the mind is the central command for the rest of the chemical actions. The output of these actions and reactions are responsible for our wellbeing, joy, happiness, enjoyment and health.

Our body is made up of billions and billions of cells. These cells require fresh oxygen to perform their daily routine work of body. If the required amount of oxygen does not reach these cells, then the toxins start accumulating around the cells and we get many complaints of headache, pain in muscles, not feeling well, etc.

Body is a unique machine; and various organs like lungs, heart, kidneys, lever, pancreas, intestines, stomach, eyes, ears, nostrils, gallbladder, and many other small organs are working with one another to give us pleasure and happiness. If any organ stops working as per the requirement, we do not feel well and we can not enjoy life. These organs are much more precious to us than furniture, jewellery, stereo-system, car, clothes, but we pay more attention to and take good care of them rather than of our body organs. How many of us have seen these valuable organs of our own body? The answer is probably 'none'. We can not see them, so we ignore them. It is said that "out of sight is out of mind". To live happy and healthy life, we must take good care of them.

For example, you have severe headache; under this condition you will not be interested in watching movies or attending any party. So the bottom line is that all your body organs should work in line and in harmony with one another to enjoy the life.

From Constipation to Cancer, Asthma to Alzheimer, all these chronic or deadly diseases are the result of the accumulation of organic waste inside the body over a period of time. These wastes are identified by science as 'toxins'. These toxins are a slow poison, and they disturb the health and functioning of the body system. Due to these disturbances, we get headache, back pain, constipation, allergies, cold, cough, and face many more problems in our everyday-life.

How are these toxins accumulated in our body? Bad habits of eating, modern life styles and lack of laborious work are the main reasons for this mess.

Proper breathing, good food eating habits, and balanced exercise will throw out these toxins from the body and stop generating these wastes inside the body.

We all know that this life looks so beautiful and pleasant by our five senses. With the help of our five senses, we live this life with full plea-sure, happiness and serenity. Theses five sense are: Touching (skin), Smelling (nose), Tasting (tongue), Seeing (eyes), and Hearing (ears).

Control of these five senses is absolutely essential to balance life and to enjoy living for many many good years. Restraint of these senses is possible only with strong will power of mind and practice of Yoga.

With this unique system, we live our life the way we should live. Happiness and enjoyment are experienced through these five senses, and they actually represent the final state of mind. It is the mind which commands these senses; and happiness is ultimately transferred into the waves of thoughts inside the mind.

The Breath:

Breathing is the most vital process of the body. It influences the activities of each and every cell and, most importantly, is intimately linked with the performance of the brain.

Human beings breathe about 15 times per minute on an average and about 22,000 times per day. Respiration fuels the burning of oxygen and glucose, producing energy to power every muscular contraction, glandular secretion and mental process. The breath is intimately linked to all aspects of human experience.

Breathing is life and life is breath. Imagine what will happen if you stop breathing for a few minutes. Breathing is a non-stop function of the body, even during sleep and unconscious state of mind.

Most of us breathe incorrectly, using only a small part of our lung capacity. Irregular and incomplete breathing disrupts the rhythms of the brain and leads to physical, emotional and mental blocks. These, in turn, lead to inner conflicts, imbalanced personality, disordered lifestyle and diseases.

Those who breath short and quick are likely to have a shorter life span than those who breath slowly and deeply. The ancient yogis and rishis in India studied the nature in great details. Animals, such as pythons, elephants and tortoises, having a slow breathing rate, have long life spans, whereas birds, dogs and rabbits, having a fast breathing rate, live for only a few years.

This is true because respiration is directly related to heart. A slow breathing rate keeps the heart strongly well nourished and contributes to a longer life span. Deep breathing also increases the absorption of energy by pranayama, enhancing dynamism, vitality and general well-being.

Pranayama establishes regular breathing patterns. Details of pranayama are discussed later.

The Mind:

"Where there is a will, there is a way". If you have strong mind power, you can accomplish any kind of task. You can even recover very fast from illness. With the power of mind, you can overcome the ups and downs of your life, very silently.

Remember the 23 years that Mr. Nelson Mandela had spent in jail. It was his power of mind that kept his body and mind healthy and fit. Mind has boundless power and abilities. We use about 10 to 20 % of the capacity of mind, on an average, during our life span. The source of both disease and healing can be found in the mind.

You can develop any and every skill you want, provided you have enough will power to learn and patience to practice. The more you try, the more you learn. For learning, mind has the sky as the limit.

Comparison between mind and computer

The human mind is often compared to a computer. In fact, we can draw an interesting analogy between a computer virus-attack and the mind being plagued by virus-like evil thoughts. The human mind, too, needs to protect itself by shoring up goodness, through right thinking and living. This will help us immunize ourselves against virus-like corrupting influences.

Like firewalls designed to protect computers from virus-attacks, the human mind, too, can institute safeguards, "firewalls" of right conduct: Non-violence in thoughts, words and deed; truthfulness and geniality of speech; absence of anger even on provocation; abstaining from malicious gossip, compassion for all creatures."

A "virus-infected" mind, in turn, severely affects the health of the body, which, in turn affects the individual's general well-being. In contrast, virtues are divine by nature and they keep mind and human body in good form.

So, like anti-virus programs designed to thwart virus-attacks in computers, we, too, have to protect ourselves from getting carried away by demonic, virus-like attributes.

Honesty, compassion, humanity and charity are virtues programmed into the human mind by God. These virtues are so natural that responding to them requires minimum or negligible Central Processing Unit utilization.

3

Food: Fuel of our Body

When we buy a new car, we try to fill up the tank with super unleaded gasoline. We take care of our car-engine with the best available fuel, but we never think about the engine of our body. We fill up our body-tank with whatever food whenever comes across our way. Time has come for us to think about what food is good and what is not. The present day diseases in modern life style are mainly caused by bad eating habits. We must ask the following five questions to introspect ourselves, and try to find their answers:

- Why should we eat?
- What should we eat?
- When should we eat?
- How much should we eat?
- How should we eat?

Our health and happiness depends on two factors: one is the food we eat and the other is our thoughts in mind when we eat. Food and mind are correlated and they act together. Food affects the body differently, depending on when and under what circumstances it is eaten.

Why should we eat?

The health-motto is: "Eat to live, rather than live to eat". It is best if we understand that the purpose of eating is to supply the life-force, or

Prana, the vital life energy. The greatest nutritional plan for the healthy and happy life is the simple diet of natural fresh foods.

We all know that body is a unique machine. This machine needs food as a source of nutrition in the form of proteins, carbohydrates, fats, minerals, and vitamins to generate energy for balanced functioning of all the organs of the body. We eat food with taste but the body system accepts it as these five nutrition contents.

We must not forget that food is fuel, not just food. Eating is making blood; exercise is distributing blood; and breathing is purifying blood.

What should we eat?

When we eat nutritional food, mind is responsible to control proper digestive process through adding of digestive enzymes in balanced quantities. To get healthy and happy, we should eat good food, and our mind should be free from any stress, tension, worries. Balanced diet includes protein, carbohydrates, fat, vitamins, minerals and water.

Can you remember what you ate last year on this date? Hardly anyone can remember except for specific events. We cannot even remember what we ate last month or a few days back. In just a few minutes, it becomes history and leaves a legacy of diseases and suffering if we have eaten wrong food.

Whatever we eat, once it enters the throat, it is simply a chemical compound of carbohydrates, protein, vitamins, etc. All those taste and overeating, due to aroma, color and taste of food, last for a few seconds as long as the food remains in our mouth.

Therefore we should eat wisely; it is fuel for body and not the taste for mouth. We must eat what our body needs and not what our mouth and tongue want. We should avoid snacking. It is a killer for our body.

Avoid red meat, fried and oily foods, chocolates and junk food. Do not smoke, drink too much tea or coffee or aerated drinks and always be conscious about white sugar. Sugar and Salt are two main killer of our life. We pay a tremendous price for not understanding this simple truth.

When should we eat?

Once we fill up our car-tank, we do not visit a gas station until it gets close to empty. The same principle applies to our body. We should skip three hours after starchy foods or protein meals, four hours after meat or heavy food, and one hour after fruit before we should eat again.

We should not eat too late at night, for there should be a gap of at least two or, preferably, three hours between dinner and sleep. Food should be freshly prepared and eaten with attention, respect and gratitude. We must be really hungry before we start eating again. Eating time should be observed with perfect punctuality.

How much should we eat?

"First serving is best, second serving is for taste and third serving is just waste"; this is the fact as said in Ayurveda. One half of our stomach should be filled with food, one fourth with water or liquid and the rest one fourth should be kept empty for gas movement during digestion. This arrangement will make digestion very smooth and will not cause any gas problem in the stomach.

The exact quantity of food we should eat depends on different parameters like work, age, location, atmosphere, weight, etc. Less food ensures healthy brain. For example, Sir Isaac Newton, when engaged in his most arduous labors, lived on bread and water, and fasted for long intervals. But one thing is sure that we must feel hungry three hours after the previous meal.

The greatest enemy of health and long life is over-eating. Over-eating is harmful in a number of ways. It may cause indigestion, promote obesity, poison the whole system, and cause a severe strain on heart, kidneys or liver.

The secret of perfect health may be summed up as a complete combustion of the fuel put into human furnace. Indeed, to be perfectly healthy, we should live in a state of almost continuous gentle hunger.

How should we eat?

How we eat food is just as important as what we eat. If we are late for work and drive in traffic, worry about getting back on time while we are eating a sandwich, our body is not going to respond the same way to the food as if we were sitting in the backyard, looking at the flowers, while we were eating.

Eating should be slow and our mind should be involved in every bite. The number of bites should be as big as possible. For example, let us take a slice of pizza. Say, we are making eight bites to finish that slice. We should finish that same slice in 13 to 15 bites. Every bite should be chewed for at least 30 to 40 times. More bites and more time for chewing the food mean food will remain in the mouth for a longer period of time. Mind will get more pleasure-feeling commands for eating food. Once the mind satisfies, we will tend to eat less food. This is the best way of dieting, controlling weight and improving health through smooth and easy digestion.

The yogic diet:

Yogic diet is a vegetarian one, consisting of pure, simple, natural foods, which digest easily and promote health. Nutritional requirements fall under five categories: protein, carbohydrates, minerals, fats and vitamins. We should have certain knowledge of dietetics in order to balance the diet. Eating foods first-hand from nature, grown in fertile soil (preferably organic, free from chemicals and pesticides), will help ensure a better supply of these nutritional needs. Processing, refining, overcooking, and complex cooking, or we can say complex food, destroy much food value and cause a burden on our digestive system.

There is a cycle, in nature, known as the "food cycle" or the "food chain". The Sun is the source of energy for all life on our planet; it nourishes the plants (the top of the food chain) which are then eaten by animals (herbivores), which are then eaten by other animals (carnivores). The food at the top of the food chain, being directly nourished by the Sun, has the greatest life promoting properties.

The food value of animal flesh is termed as the "second-hand" source of nutrition, and is inferior in nature. All natural foods (fruits, vegetables, seeds, nuts and grains) have, in varying quantities, different proportions of these essential nutrients. As a source of protein, these are easily assimilated by the body. However, the second-hand sources are often more difficult to digest and are of less value to the body's metabolism.

Many people worry whether or not they are getting enough protein, but they neglect other factors. The quality of protein is more important than the quantity alone. Dairy products, legumes, nuts and seeds provide the vegetarian with an adequate supply of protein.

However, the true Yogic diet is actually more selective than this. A Yogi is concerned with the subtle effect that the food has on his mind and astral body. He therefore avoids foods which are overly stimulating, preferring those which render the mind calm and the intellect sharp.

Any change in diet should be made gradually. We should start by substituting larger portions of vegetables, grains, seeds and nuts until finally all flesh products have been completely eliminated from the diet.

The Yogic diet will help us attain a high standard of health, keen intellect and serenity of mind. To understand truly the Yogic approach to diet, we have to get familiar with the concept of the three Gunas or qualities of nature.

Any dog or horse-trainer will tell us that what is fed to an animal influences its behavior. Although we like to forget this when it comes to ourselves, what we eat has a huge influence not only over our physical well being, but also over our thoughts and, ultimately, our emotional and spiritual well-being. However, proper diet is a controversial subject.

Nutrition has been extensively researched by modern science, and there seems to be as many 'proper' diets as there are scientific studies. It is more than a bit confusing for someone to devise his own individual diet amidst so much, often contradictory, advice. The advice given below is based on the classical yogic texts and on my personal experience.

Unlike modern scientists, yogis are less interested in the chemical content (protein, vitamins, etc…) of the food. According to their practice, food is traditionally classified to its effect on the body and mind, using the three Gunas: **Sattva** (the quality of love, light and life), **Raja** (the quality of activity and passion, but lacking stability) and **Tamas** (the quality of darkness and inertia, dragging us into ignorance and attachment).

Sattvic (Nutrition) food promotes clarity and calmness of mind and is favorable for spiritual growth. It is "sweet, fresh and agreeable" and includes most fruits, nuts, seeds, vegetables, particularly green leafy vegetables, whole grains, honey, pure water and milk (with the reservation that commercially produced milk may not nowadays be so sattvic…). Given the amount of pesticides and chemical fertilizers used on commercial crops, only organic products still qualify as Sattvic, and tinned or frozen foods certainly do not.

Rajasic (Neutral) food feeds the body, promotes activity and therefore induces restlessness of mind. It disturbs the equilibrium of the mind and is generally to be avoided by yoga practiceners. Rajasic foods include most spicy foods; stimulants like coffee and tea; eggs, garlic, onion, meat, fish and chocolate, as well as most of the processed foods. Eating too fast or with a disturbed mind is also considered Rajasic. Rajasic food should be avoided by those whose aim is to get peace of mind, but it will benefit people with an active lifestyle. A little Rajasic food can be sattvic. For example, hot spices can help digestion, and therefore help create peace of mind!

Tamasic food (to be avoided) induces heaviness of the body and dullness of the mind, and ultimately benefits neither. It includes alcohol, as well as food that are stale or overripe. Overeating is also tamasic. The traditional advice is to fill the stomach half with food, one quarter with water, leaving the last quarter empty for gas movement in the stomach.

The nature of food can change the type of preparing food. Cooking is the most obvious way to change the nature of food. Grains become sattvic only after cooking. Honey becomes tamasic (poisonous) with cooking. The nature of food also changes by being in combination with other foods and spices, or if it is stored for a long period of time. Generally, grains should be aged a bit (they become more sattvic) but, of course, fruits shouldn't be (they rot and become tamasic).

Ayurveda opines that the fear of death permeate every cell of the body of an animal when it is slaughtered, and, therefore, the traditional yogic diet is lacto-vegetarian; it avoids eggs as well as all animal flesh (including fish!). Indeed, modern research has shown that vegetarians are generally in better health than meat-eaters in the long run and in the later years of life.

Proteins that can be obtained from nuts, dairy products, beans and legumes are generally of a better quality than meat. Anyone who has lived for a while on a dairy farm might go as far as questioning the morality of eating dairy products when the milk is taken from a cow whose calf has been taken away and slaughtered.

Another important point to consider is how any particular diet suits an individual's particular constitution and circumstances.

Food Combining:

By understanding the basic process of food digestion, it is now clear by practice that body cannot cope with protein (meat, fish, poultry etc.) and carbohydrates (bread, rice, potatoes) in the same meal because they fight and cannot be properly digested. Incompletely digested food is said to be difficult to eliminate, causing weight gain and toxicity in the cells and tissues.

Eating the two types of food together is said to lead to the overproduction of acid in the stomach. Oil, Butter, Margarine, Herbs, and Spices are neutral and can be combined with any food. Fruits must be eaten in isolation.

Finally, the issue of food combining, which has received some attention in the West in recent years, is also important, for even the right foods taken in wrong combination can cause problems. Without going into too much detail, let us just say that some types of food combine well, while others should not be mixed because of the difference in their digestive processes.

For example, strong proteins should not be mixed with carbohydrates. To be safe, avoid mixing too many different types of food in the same meal. There are many more approaches to dieting. Eating the right food, in the right amount, in the right combination, at the right time, is a difficult art, which can only be learned by experimenting to find out what works best for you.

Water: An Elixir of Life

65% of our body is made of water and also with the help of water. Water is the most essential part of our whole body system of blood, cells, tissues, organs, bones, etc. Due to this fact, we must maintain water level inside our body for smooth operation of all activities.

Do not wait until you get thirsty. You should drink at least ten glasses of water per day. Studies have shown that a decrease in water intake will cause fat deposits to increase; while an increase in water intake can actually reduce fat deposits.

The kidney cannot function properly without enough water. Water can help relieve constipation. When the body gets too little water, it siphons what it needs from the internal sources. The colon is the one primary source. Results? Constipation. But when a person drinks enough water, normal bowel function usually returns. Water helps to get rid of the waste from the body.

During weight loss, the body has a lot more waste to get rid of—all that metabolized fat will be shed. An overweight person needs more water than a thin one. Water should be pure and free from any residue or excessive amount of minerals.

Timing of drinking water: Take 2 to 4 glasses of luke-warm water as soon as you get up in the early morning. For the whole night your digestive track system has been empty as no food has been taken for last 6 to 8 hours. When you drink luke-warm water in the morning, this starts cleaning the inside walls of your bowels, washes out anything left inside the stomach and gets rid of any kind of constipation for ever. Daily habit of this early drinking water gives unbelievable results for no cost.

Avoid water for one hour before and after taking any breakfast, lunch and dinner. Our digestive system gets ready for food intake at proper time, and water, before and after food, will dilute the digestive enzymes.

Cold water or Hot water? The inside temperature of our body is around 98.4 degree F. When we drink cold water from a freeze, it disturbs the inside body temperature, causing an upset in the digestive process. For drinking purpose, normal or slight cold water is perfect.

For the purpose of taking a bath or shower, luke-warm water is the best. Too much hot water makes bones stiff and after bath we feel lazy rather than fresh and energetic.

Unique Herbal Juice:

Every morning you should take the herbal juice in the quantity of about 4 to 5 teaspoonfuls. Take small pieces of Ginger and Turmeric (both fresh) and one Amala (English name is Phyllenthus emblica), all available in Indian grocery stores. (If an Amala is not available, then use a few drops of fresh lemon juice). Extract juices from these three herbals. Add one spoonful of honey to these. Drink this mixed juice after 45 to 60 minutes of morning water-intake, every day.

Note: If you are underweight or do not want to reduce the weight, then do not add honey to this juice. Honey, when mixed with Amala or lemon juice, reduces the weight.

This is unique in the sense that it reduces the weight without any fatigue and side effects, cleans the lungs of cough, eases from bronchitis, purifies the blood, brightens the skin, balances appetite, and removes the black spots on the skin.

A Day with Liquid Food Only:

This is the best way to clean up the inner toxins and waste from the body. Spend the whole day or half day, beginning with only liquid food.

Start the day with 2 to 4 glasses of luke-warm water. Then go for herbal juice as discussed earlier. Vegetable soup, lemon juice, orange juice, fresh fruit juice, butter milk or coconut water are a few, best liquid drinks.

Because there is no solid food in the digestive track, the whole system would get a necessary break, and the drink will clean the entire digestive system and body of toxins collected in cells.

Food and Fibre:

Dietary fibre has been a hot news item in the recent decade. Man always has a tendency to choose tasty and highly refined food which has instant pleasure value. But the fact is that almost all the diseases of modern civilization are attributed to the processing of foods and the reduced intake of fibrous foods.

Fibre is an important element of some foods of plant origin. Fibre is of two types—soluble and insoluble. Insoluble fibre does not dissolve in water, is bulky and passes through the digestive system quickly. Soluble fibre dissolves in water and passes through the digestive tract slowly.

A lack of fibre in the diet has been associated with several gastro-intestinal disorders, including constipation, diseases of the colon and even colon cancer. In addition, fibre-deficient diet has been associated with several metabolic disorders such as diabetes, obesity, arthritis, and many others.

High-fibre foods may be of particular help to people with obesity. They are usually low in calories, increase the satisfaction, thus preventing excess intake of food. It is also helpful in the treatment of diabetes. Fibre in the diet delays the absorption of sugar, thus preventing the rapid rise of post-meal blood sugar.

High fibre foods are in plenty: raw unprocessed fruits and vegetables, nuts, pulses, whole grains, oat-meals and beans. A daily fibre intake of about 30-40 grams is adequate. Eat whole grain foods with their natural fibrous coatings (husk), e. g. whole wheat flour, and whole wheat bread in place of white bread. Eat whole, fresh fruits with their peels (whenever possible) instead of fruit juices. Amala, apple, grapes, pineapple, blackberry, orange, gooseberry, watermelon, peach, pawpaw, jackfruit, strawberry are the best rich fruits in fibre. Make sprouted beans, green leafy vegetables and raw salads a part of your daily diet. Vegetables with high fibre content are beetroot, carrot, tomato, radish, yam, potato, sweet potato, french beans, capsicum, and spinach.

Drink 10 glasses of water a day since fibre draws water into your intestine and passes easily through the intestine. Increase the amount of dietary fibre slowly over a period of time. Remember that adding too much of fibre too quickly can cause stomach upsets.

Food, Fever and Fast:

When the body gets fever, our immune system is fighting against outside viruses or bacteria. Due to this fighting, our body temperature rises. We should not get panicked. Rather, we must cooperate with our immune system so that it can safeguard our body.

First thing we should do under this circumstance is to stop eating fried, fatty and other complex foods. If possible, we should go for liquid food. The best remedy is to fast for a day or two. Fasting is the best bet in case of fever. When there is no food in stomach, our immune system utilizes all its energy to fight with the outside forces.

As the body requires cleaning during illness, the mind needs to be periodically cleansed, and we must try to maintain it in a state of purity. The mind-body theory vindicates the benefits of fasting. Fasting increases our powers of concentration, improves our mental as well as spiritual strength, and gives peace of mind, confidence and courage.

It is well known that Jesus, Moses, Buddha and almost all the ancient sages of India abstained from food at various times in courses of their pursuits of spiritual insight and purification.

Fresh Fruits and Green Vegetables:

Fresh fruits and green vegetables should be considered an essential part of diet. They are Mother Nature's best gift to us. Their nutritional values protect us from many deadly diseases.

Rainbow revolution should be the part of daily eating pattern. Fruits and vegetables of seven different colors should be included in our dish every day.

Look at the different eye-catching colors of Bits, Orange, Strawberry, green leafy vegetables, Banana etc. Their colors inspire you to eat them. Make a habit of eating them every day.

Veg or Non-Veg:

Nowadays almost everyone is confused about whether or not vegetarian diet is good for health or non-veg diet is ok. There are many people who are strictly vegetarian but hardly we can find anyone who is only non-veg. We get approximately 60 to 70 % our nutrition value from our vegetarian foods.

Animals or any other living creatures get frightened when they realize their slaughter. This situation produces toxins inside their system due to abrupt changes in mind. This is true for any living organism including human beings.

These toxins, preserved for a long time between slaughter and serving, make the non-veg food unfit for health. It develops much complication in the body's immune system. Non-veg food is just for taste and waste, and it is not good for our body in the modern life style.

Many argue that if non-veg food is totally stopped, then there will be shortage of food in the world. This is not true because animals require a lot of land and water to survive. They also produce pollution, whereas plants and trees are the best environment-friendly agents, and are helpful in purifying the air.

Vegetarian foods are easy to digest, compared to non-veg food. In case of any digestive disorder, non-veg foods are more likely to develop toxins in blood.

Eat Less, Live long: A true story of Louie Cornerro

This is a true story of Mr. Louie Cornerro born around the 15th century, in a rich Italian family. He was born weak on account of a luxurious life style in a rich family. He was a victim of many diseases before his 40th birth day. Many doctors tried many medicines on his body but they did not work at all. Sometimes he thought of committing suicide because of this sickness and the resultant depression.

One day, he found out that thin people, living with discipline, could live longer. On the other hand, healthy people, living unwisely, died early. So he firmly decided to live with control and discipline. He realized that, to save himself from death and disease, this was the only way left to him.

Many people believe that the food they like is good for their body and health but Mr. Louie found that it was totally wrong. He did stop eating cold wines, fish, meat, sweets, fried and oily food. After many days of experiment, he found out which food was good for his stomach. He also started eating in less quantity, even though he wanted to eat more. For the next one year, he ate simple food in less quantity. Soon he became free from all types of diseases. He became healthier than he was in his young age. He regained his original health and became stronger.

Mr. Louie Cornerro had lived for 100 years. He wrote four articles on his life and experiments. The first article he wrote at the age of 83, the second at the age of 86, the third at the age of 91 and the fourth (in the form of letters to his friend) at the age of 95.

The importance of this story is not that he lived for 100 years, but he was born weak and almost recovered from all the diseases before he was forty years old. Moderate quantity of plain and simple food gave him a prolonged life. Always leave the dinning table while you are still a little hungry, to avoid over-eating. This is something we should observe and practice in our life everyday.

Food and nutrition:

Nutrition begins with food. The science of nutrition concerns everything that the body does with food in order for it to sustain, grow, function and heal.

Foods eaten on a regular basis make up a diet. Although geographic locations and family traditions play major roles in forming dietary habits, food choices vary from person to person. To a high degree, what people eat affects their health, their enjoyment of life and longevity. In turn, healthy habits and a happy outlook can improve the ways in which the human body makes use of food. With the help of the sun, plants get their food from chemicals in the earth, water, and air.

Calories

The body's most basic need is energy. To get energy, it needs food as a fuel, and oxygen to burn it. The amount of energy the foods produce is measured in units called calories. A food calorie, or a kilocalorie, is the amount of heat required to raise the temperature of 1 kilogram (2.2 pounds) of water to 1 degree Celsius (1.8 degrees Fahrenheit).

Energy Needs

The body converts the calories in food into energy, which is necessary for every act, from blinking an eye to running a race. Energy is also used for the process of growing, for rebuilding damaged cells, and for regulating body systems.

The number of calories needed each day depends upon how much energy an individual's body uses. An active child needs more calories than an adult who works at a desk. The body needs more calories in cold weather in order to stay at an even temperature.

Stored Energy

If a person takes in more food than required to meet the body's needs, the excess calories are converted to fat-a stored form of energy. That causes weight gain. Eating too little causes weight loss because the stored fat is used up for energy. One pound (0.5 kilogram) of stored fat contains about 3,500 calories.

If a weight loss is advisable, the best way to lose is to eat less food of high-calorie values and do more exercise. For most people a safe limit for losing weight is 2 pounds a week.

Nutrients

To function, the human body must have nutrients. The essential nutrients for human beings are proteins, carbohydrates, fats/oils, minerals, vitamins, and water.

Proteins (15 to 20%)

Proteins are made of amino acids, small units necessary for growth and tissue repair. Protein is body's most essential substance, along with water and fat. Animal foods such as meat, fish, poultry, milk, and eggs are rich in protein. Beans, peas, nuts, bread, and cereals are very good plant sources of protein.

Combining plant sources, such as peanut butter with whole-grain bread, or rice with beans, provides excellent protein rich food. So does

combining plant and animal sources such as cereal and milk, or maca-
roni and cheese.

Carbohydrates (40 to 50%)

Starches and sugars are carbohydrates, the main source of the body's
energy. Carbohydrates account for about half of the calorie intake by
most Americans and up to four fifths of the calories in diets of Africans
and Asians. Carbohydrate-rich foods are also the main sources of protein for most of the people in the world. Rice, wheat, corn, and potatoes are common rich sources of carbohydrates.

Sugars are not essential foods. They provide energy (calories) but no
nutrients. For that reason sugar is called an "empty calorie" food.
Occasional sweets are not harmful to a healthy, active person, but
excessive sugar can lead to tooth decay when sticky snack foods that
cling to teeth are eaten between meals.

Fats and Oils (3 to 5%)

Fats and oils (which are liquid) are a concentrated source of energy.
Fats in the diet are necessary for good health. They make certain vitamins for use in the body; they cushion vital organs; they make up a
part of all body cells; and they help to maintain body temperature. Fats
also delay pangs of hunger because a food mixture containing fat
remains longer in the stomach.

Minerals

Minerals are neutral elements. They are inorganic. Almost all foods
contribute to a varied intake of essential minerals. Most minerals are
easy to obtain in quantities required by the body. A major exception is
iron for children under the age of 4, adolescent girls, and women in the
childbearing years. These groups need more iron than a normal diet
may provide. Iron helps to build red blood cells. It also helps the blood

to carry oxygen from the lungs to each body cell. Rich sources of iron are egg plants and dark, green vegetables.

Everyone at every age needs calcium. This mineral builds bones and teeth, and it is necessary for blood clotting. The best sources are milk and hard cheese. Others are leafy greens, nuts, and small fishes—such as sardines—with bones that can be eaten.

Phosphorus works with calcium to make strong bones and teeth. A diet that furnishes enough protein and calcium also provides enough phosphorus. Other important minerals are sodium, potassium, iodine, magnesium, zinc, and copper.

Vitamins

The discovery of vitamins began early in the 20th century. It is likely that some are still undiscovered. Eating a wide variety of foods ensures getting enough vitamins whether or not they are identified. All living things need vitamins for growth and health. The body cannot normally manufacture them either at all or in sufficient amount, and so they must be obtained from food. Each vitamin has specific roles to play. Many reactions in the body require several vitamins, and the lack or excess of anyone can interfere with the normal function of the body system.

Fat-soluble vitamins

Four vitamins—A, D, E, and K—are known as the fat-soluble vitamins. They are digested and absorbed with the help of fats in the diet.

Vitamin A is needed for strong bones, good vision, and healthy skin. It is found both in dark, green and in yellow fruits and vegetables.

Vitamin D is essential for children because it helps calcium and phosphorus to form straight, strong bones and teeth. With direct sunlight on the skin, the body can manufacture its own vitamin D. Infants and young children often need a vitamin D supplement. Vitamin D is added routinely to most milk during processing. Morning sun rays are a good source of these vitamins

<u>Vitamin E</u> helps to protect vitamin A and red blood cells. It is found in a wide variety of foods, and almost everyone gets it enough.

<u>Vitamin K</u> is one vitamin that is made by bacteria within the human body. They live in the intestinal tract. Small amounts of this vitamin are found in the green leaves of spinach, kale, cabbage, and cauliflower and also in pork liver.

Fat-soluble vitamins can be stored in the body for long periods. They are stored mostly in the fatty tissues and in the liver.

Water-soluble vitamins

The vitamin B group of several vitamins helps to maintain healthy skin and well-functioning of the nervous system. Vitamin B also helps to convert carbohydrates into energy.

Vitamin C, or ascorbic acid, is needed for building the connective tissues that hold body cells together. Vitamin C is essential for healthy teeth, gums, and blood vessels. It also helps the body to absorb iron. These water-soluble vitamins are not stored in the body for long. Food with this group of vitamins should be eaten every day.

Water

In order to live, every cell in the body must be bathed in water. Water takes an active part in many chemical reactions, and is needed to carry other nutrients to body organs, to regulate body temperature, and to help eliminate wastes. Water makes up about 65 percent of an adult's body weight. Requirements for water are met in many ways. Most fruits contain more than 90 percent of water.

Balanced Food

For most of us, balanced food means proteins, carbohydrates, fats, minerals and vitamins in proper proportion. When we talk about balanced food, then it means food from varieties of sources of all essential elements required for the body.

We should eat different types of food in each category. There are many types of grains; pulses and beans; fruits; vegetables; herbals and spices.

Grains: Wheat, Rice, Oat, Millet, Maize, Barley, etc.

Pulses and Beans: Kidney beans, Cluster beans, Peas, Lentils, Gram, Phaseolies mungo, Lima beans, Soya beans, Runner beans, Wax beans, Stick beans, Ground nuts, etc.

Fruits: Apple, Pineapple, Guava, Pomegranate, Grapes, Fig, Peach, Plum, Banana, Pawpaw, Strawberry, Blackberry, Mulberry, Litchis, Orange, Waternut, Cherry, Watermelon, Almond, Cashewnut, Walnut, Dates, Jackfruit, Sapodilla, Coconut, Custard apple, Avocado, Grapefruit, Apricot, etc.

Vegetables: Cauliflower, Radishes, Carrots, Egg Plant, Potatoes, Onions, Cabbage, Lettuce, Spinach, Beetroot, Broccoli, Cucumber, Pumpkin, Asparagus, Sugar beet, Bell pepper, Marrows, Tomatoes, Celery, Parsley, Fenugreek, Okra, Tinda, Drumstick, Sweet Potatoes, Yam, Elephant's foot, Mushrooms, Snake gourd, Bitter gourd, Bottle gourd, Striped pear gourd, Turnip, Arum, Lemon, etc.

Herbals and spices: Turmeric, Garlic, Ginger, Dry Ginger, Chilly, Capsicum, Coriander seeds and leaves, Basil leaves, Caraway, Black pepper, Asafetida, Clove, Niger or Seasamum, Cinnamon, Nutmeg, Cumin seeds, Saffron, Camphor, Phyllenthus emblica, Myrobalan, Fennel seeds, Dry date, Cardamom, Buck wheat, Mustard, Castor seed, Honey, Tamarind, Menthol, etc.

How many of us eat any of the above foods once in a month? These foods are good for body and should be part of our daily diet according to their availability in a season. Most of the fruits and vegetables are available in certain parts of the year and they are best to eat them in that season. We must create rainbow revolution in our daily dishes. Different kinds of colorful foods should be on our eating menu.

Food and Power of Mind

Digestive process and mind are related to each other. You must first educate and prepare your mind to enforce any regulation about diet. Cooperation of mind is required when you decide to avoid a particular food which you like most.

The more you suppress the mind to avoid the food, the more it will force you in future to eat that delicious food. Slowly and steadily, with the help of the mind, start your particular diet, with full confidence and dedication. The gospel for healthy body: We should eat to live, not live to eat.

4

Obesity: Mother of all diseases

Until now obesity was considered the disorder of the body, but no more so now. Obesity is now considered a disease. It is the source of many diseases of modern life style, like hypertension, heart attack, diabetes, arthritis, asthma, indigestion, acidity, any many more. The list is endless.

Following are the main reasons why obesity in human bodies is seen in people of all ages, all over the world:

- Lack of knowledge and will power to live a happy and healthy life,
- Stress and tension in life,
- Eating considered a fun and pleasure,
- Eating a lot of food at parties, in the company of like minded friends and families,
- No exercise and no labor intensive work in daily life,
- Eating a lot of junk foods,
- Frequent eating.

As per a research report, obesity reduces 25% of our life span. Obesity is more dangerous than any other single disease, and is considered a main killer nowadays.

Obesity can be reduced and controlled very easily if a person has enough will power. Following are the easy steps to control obesity.

- Do for 15 to 30 minutes some aerobic exercises of your choice, where your heart beats become double and you are sweating even in winter. Sport is the best to reduce excess weight. Tennis, Badminton, Basketball, Football are considered best sport for this purpose. When you play sports in group, chances are that you will not be bored and tired.

- Add low calories of food to your diet. By eating certain foods, you may feel you have eaten a lot of food but the body receives only a few calories.

- Fruit juices and leafy vegetables should be taken in considerable amount in regular diet.

- Eat only when you become really hungry.

- Fasting is also a good try to reduce weight. Try to remain only on liquid food for a half or full day, at times.

What is the ideal weight?

The weight of a person varies according to his height. Your weight should be proportionate to your height in inches. If you are 5'5" tall, then your ideal weight should be 65 kg., One kilogram of weight per inch of your body-height. A margin of 5% plus or minus is considered reasonable.

Obesity and Longevity

Obesity and Longevity are acting in opposite direction. As obesity increases, longevity decreases, and vice versa. Even if you are healthy and have no disease in your early age, you may cut short your life span due to obesity. Due to obesity, veins come under severe pressure and this affects blood circulation. Blood flow in certain micro veins become standstill, resulting in paralytic attack. Due to increase of cholesterol level in blood, circulation to vital organs of body like brain is disturbed. Brain hemorrhage and heart attack take place without notice. It has been proved that the lean live long. The person who is lean and slim has more chances to live a longer life without any disease.

Obesity: a disease nobody desires

Obesity is now considered a disease and not just a disorder. It is a life style disease and it has nothing to do with any virus or bacteria. It is simply due to lack of understanding and knowledge of the functioning of the body and its organs. Here is a special but simple yoga asana which is very useful in burning excess fat deposited around the waist and on buttocks. It is a very good asana for women who want slim waistlines.

Yoga Asana to reduce weight:

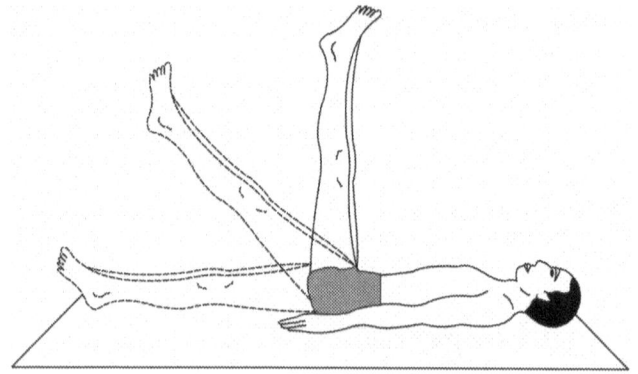

Position:

- Lie down on a blanket, with face upward.
- Keep both hands beside the body, with palms to the floor.

- Close the eyes and relax the whole body for a few seconds.
- Slowly lift both the legs together and hold at a 30 degree angle. Count 1 to 15.
- Then again raise the legs to a 60 degree angle and count 1 to 15.
- Then raise the legs up to a 90 degree angle and count 1 to 15.
- After counting 15, bring back both the legs to a 60 degree angle and then 30 degree angle. Slowly bring the legs down on the floor. Relax for one minute and repeat the cycle again.
- Observe the pain while holding the legs at 30, 60 and 90 degree levels. Concentrate the mind on the movement of the legs.
- Both the legs should be lifted and brought down together.

Benefits:

Extra fat deposited around waist and buttocks start burning while holding the legs at different angles. The pain you feel is due to burning of calories in the form of fat. The body will get slimed at the waistline. Patience and practice are required to get the results.

5

Yoga: An Introduction

Whenever we hear the word Yoga, different thoughts and imaginations come to our mind. Usually we think that Yoga is only for the rich; Yoga takes a lot of time; Yoga is difficult to do; etc. As a truth, all our above assumptions are wrong. Yoga is simple to do, it takes very little time and it is for anyone who wants to live long, healthy and happy life.

Yoga is derived from the Sanskrit root 'Yuj', meaning "to unite", "to integrate" or "to cohere" and is thus taken to represent the highest state of union, integration or coherence between individual or personal or human consciousness and cosmic or universal or divine consciousness.

Yoga is that extraordinary, exemplary, unique Indian technique, helping man to develop a deep awareness by himself of every vibration and pulsation within—at the body, mind and intellect levels, by virtue of which he can master the forces of the internal and the external.

Yoga is a spiritual science of self-realization. Yoga is the science of holistic living. Yoga is the science of activating your inner energies in such a way that your body, mind and emotions function at their highest peak. Yoga means to be in perfect tune. Your body, mind, spirit and existence are in absolute harmony. When you fine-tune yourself to such a point where everything functions beautifully within you, the best of your abilities will just flow out of you. It works on all aspects of the person: physical, vital, mental, emotional, psychic and spiritual.

Yoga methods encompass the entire field of our existence, from the physical, emotional and mental to the spiritual. Its methods include ethical disciplines, physical postures; Yoga is a means of balancing and harmonizing the body, breath, mind and emotions.

Doing yoga on a regular basis gives the body a chance to break the habit of being sluggish and stiff. Glands, nervous system, heart and intestines are affected and kept flexible or restored and activated.

Unlike a cat which stretches instinctively, we learn to do it consciously. The resulting experience prompts us to continue and use yoga according to our needs and the way we live.

Yoga bestows inner strength, sharpens our intellect, teaches us to control our emotions and brings a rare concentration and efficiency into our actions and work, making one do the right thing in the right way at the right time; and that is why Yoga is often described as a skill in action. Integration and harmony should be between thought, word and deed or integration between head, heart and hand.

Swami Vivekananda condensed the entire basis, essence and streams of Yoga in a single proclamation. "Each soul is potentially divine. The goal is to manifest this divinity within, by controlling nature, external and internal. Do this either by work, or worship or psychic control or philosophy by one or more, or all of these and be free. This is the whole of religion. Doctrines or dogmas or rituals or books, or temples or forms, are but secondary details".

Yoga: Eight stages of process

It comes from India and goes back to over five thousand years. The Indian sage, Patanjali, in his Yoga sutras, defines yoga as the control of the activities of the mind, breath control, yogic diet as well as meditation. Classical yoga as defined by Patanjali is an eight-stage process of spiritual development.

The first two stages are ethical disciplines (Yamas and Nyamas). Then come postures (Asanas in Sanskrit) and breathing exercises (Pranayama). The last four limbs are meditative stages: control of the sense (Prathyara), concentration (Dharana), meditation (Dhyana) and the spiritual enlightenment (Samadhi).

The regular practice of asanas, and breathing exercises (pranayama), makes the body strong, supple and healthy. It has a profound effect on the circulation of blood and on the functioning of the inner organs, glands and nerves, keeping all systems in radiant health and leading to greater energy, better concentration, and a happier, more fulfilling life. Many common physical ailments can also be cured through the regular practice of yoga; and it is never too late or too early in life to take it up. Anyone can practice yoga and achieve wonderful results to live happy and healthy.

The science of yoga begins to work on the outermost aspect of the personality, the physical body, which, for most of the people, is a practical and familiar starting point. When imbalance is experienced at this level, the organs, muscles and nerves no longer function in harmony; rather they act in opposition to each other. As a result, the endocrine system might become irregular and the efficiency of the nervous system decrease to such an extent that a disease will manifest. Yoga aims to bring the different bodily functions into perfect coordination so that they work for the good of the whole body. When your body and mind function in a completely different state of relaxation and a certain level of bliss, you can not be released from most of suffering.

Yoga is not an exercise; it is not a pranayama; it is not even a meditation; it is a complete way of life. Yoga teaches us how to live the life with full pleasure and happiness. Yoga keeps us in present moments rather than in past or future.

Looking at the present world, we hardly live in present moments. We remain either in past or future of our life. Both states of life bring worries, anxiety, depression, mood swing, which make us unhappy and unhealthy. We can bring joy in our life only when we are living our life from moments to moments in present situation. Present time is the real life; past and future are just the memories and imaginations, respectively.

Yoga helps us to achieve that goal. Yoga is a tool to find ultimate expression and enjoyment to life. The only condition is that it must be a consistent and continuous process with full awareness.

Yoga is mainly divided into four parts as below. Each works differently but it has profound effects on others. They are all inter-connected with each other:

- Exercise (Asana)
- Breathing (Pranayama)
- Relaxation
- Meditation

Law of Least Effort:

Nature's intelligence functions with effortless ease, and when we harness the forces of harmony, joy and love, we create success and good fortune with effortless ease. If we observe nature at work, we see how little effort is expended in accomplishing wondrous tasks. The grass just grows, without trying to grow; and the fish just swim, they do not try to swim.

It is the nature of the sun to shine, and the nature of the stars to glitter and twinkle. And hence let us accept that it is the human nature to make the dream manifest into physical form easily and effortlessly. When we are in harmony with nature, when we are established in the knowledge of our true self; we can make use of the Law of Least Effort or Sahaj Bhaav.

Minimum effort is expended when our actions are motivated by love, because all of nature is held together by the energy of love. Our energy multiplies and accumulates; and the surplus energy we thus gather in the process can be channeled to create anything we want, including unlimited wealth.

If the focal point is man's ego, our attention consumes much more energy, and so is the case when we seek power and control over other people without a ray of sympathy and love; but when our internal reference point is the spirit (Self), we become immune to criticism and we are unfearful of any challenge. We can thus harness the power of love, and use energy creatively to evolve ourselves mentally and spiritually, even while succeeding in the material world.

Acceptance is the first step in this kind of Yoga. This kind of yoga is known as Sahaj Yoga or yoga with ease, without any force or compulsion. Acceptance simply means that we accept people, situations, circumstances and events as they occur—accepting every moment as it should be, because the whole universe is as it should be.

This moment—the one we are experiencing right now—is the culmination of all the moments we have experienced in the past. This moment is as it is because the whole universe is as it is. When we struggle against the moment, we are actually against the universe. This means that when our acceptance of this moment is total and complete, we shall not be struggling against the universe. It is important to understand that we need to accept the things as they are, not as we wish them to be. When we feel frustrated or upset by a person or a situation, let us remember we are not reacting to the person or situation, but to our own feelings, and our feelings are not someone else's fault.

Responsibility is the second component of the Law of Least Effort. Responsibility means not blaming anyone or anything for our situation, including ourselves. One can have a creative response to the situation as it is now. All problems contain the seeds of new opportunities, and once we develop this attitude, every so called upsetting situation will become an opportunity for the creation of something new and beautiful, and every so called tormentor or tyrant will become our teacher. If we interpret the reality in this manner, all such situations and people will be reminding us that "this moment is as it should be". There is a hidden meaning behind all events, and the hidden meaning points to our own evolution.

Defenselessness is the third component of the Law of Least Effort, which consist in relinquishing our need to convince or persuade others of our point of view. If we look around, we will see 99 % of the people persisting in defending their point of view. And if we desist from this course, we shall gain access to an enormous amount of energy that is wasted whenever we become defensive, blame others and do not accept the present. By accepting the situation, we are fully experiencing the present, which is the gift of God. When we posses this rare combination of acceptance, responsibility and defenselessness, we shall experience the life flowing with effortless ease.

6

Yogasana: To Balance the Body

The Yogic physical exercises are called Asanas, a term which means a steady posture that coordinate mind and muscles. Yog Asana (or posture) is meant to be held for some time, observing pains and feelings at certain points of body, and to increase body flexibility.

The body is as young as it is flexible. Yoga exercises focus on the health of the spine, its strength and flexibility. The spinal column houses the most important nervous system, the telegraphic system of the body. By maintaining the spine's flexibility and strength through exercise, circulation is increased and the nerves are ensured supply of their nutrients and oxygen. The Asanas also affect the internal organs and the endocrine system (glands and hormones).

Traditional exercise is goal-oriented: "How many push ups can I do? Can I touch my toes? I'm going to do 10 more crunches today than I did yesterday". Yogasanas, by contrast, is a continuous process. The idea is to focus your awareness on what you are doing and how you are feeling as you perform the postures. In a physical exercise, you fail if you miss your goal. In Yoga, you succeed by trying. There is also a difference at the physical level. Weight training, for example, makes you stronger by breaking down and rebuilding muscle tissues. It is this breaking down and rebuilding that result in the bulky muscle look. Yoga increases strength by toning the muscles.

Although there are many Asanas (8,400,000 according to the scriptures), the practice of the 20 or so basic postures brings out the essence, and provides all major benefits of this wonderful system. The asanas are divided, basically into five categories according to their purpose, position and postures.

1. Standing position asanas

2. Sitting Position asanas

3. Lying down position asanas

4. Relaxation asanas

5. Special asanas

Every category has five to eight asanas. Altogether we consider 20 asanas, which are easy to do and which affect our body and mind greatly.

Sitting Position Asanas:

1. Sukhasana (easy pose)

2. Vajrasana (Thunderbolt pose)

3. Shashankasana (pose of moon)

4. Gomukhasana (Cow's face pose)

5. Wakrasana (spinal twist pose)

6. Padmasana (lotus pose)

7. Yogamudrasana (Psychic union pose)

8. Titali (butterfly pose)

Standing Position Asanas:

9. Padahasthasana (Hand to foot Pose)

10. Paschimothanasana (Forward bend)

11. Trikonasana (Triangle Pose)

12. Tadasana (Palm Tree pose)

Lying down Position Asanas:

13. Bhujangasana (Cobra Pose)

14. Naukasana (Boat pose)

15. Dhanurasana (Bow pose)

16. Shalabhasana (Locust pose)

Relaxation Asanas:

17. Makarasana (Crocodile pose)

18. Shavasana (Dead body pose)

Special Asanas:

19. Sirshasana (Headstand Pose)

20. Sarvangasana (Shoulder stand Pose)

If we look very closely, a human being has natural tendency to do the asanas, but he does not recognize it. Our body gets stiff after our sitting at one place for a long period of time or after our getting up from sleep, or after working on one task with deep concentration. We remove this stiffness by stretching our body. During these stretching and twisting, we do the asanas without our knowledge of them. In a way, this stretching and twisting of our body is a kind of asanas.

Even animals and birds are doing this exercise. Look closely at your house-pets. When they get up from sleep or rest, they also do the asanas.

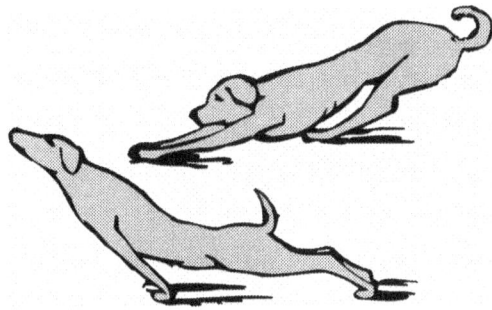

The above pictures can tell us how the animals relieve their stiffness in muscles and joints by stretching and twisting their body.

Preparing for practicing the asanas:

- Asanas are not an exercise. Asanas should be done in a slow and steady motion.

- Speed and force has no place in doing asanas. Every step should be taken gradually and smoothly.

- While doing asanas, the mind should be focused on muscles, where you can feel pain, strain or sensation. Remember that mind and muscles are correlated and they are going together.

- Presence of mind is very important while practicing asanas. If the mind is absent, benefits will be reduced to 50%.

- Avoid practicing asanas when you have fever or any other body or health problems.

- They should be done on empty stomach. They are strictly prohibited after taking lunch or dinner, unless and otherwise instructed to do so.

- Breathing pattern should be maintained as per instructions, for each asana.

- Best time to do most of the asanas is early morning when the stomach is empty and the atmosphere is cool and calm. Some asanas can be practiced at any time of the day.

- Wear loose and less clothes as far as possible for comfort in doing asanas.

- During asanas, count the numbers for time estimate and concentration.

- Never try to reach the final position by force or extra stretch or strain on muscles. Stretch the muscles up to your bearable limit. Stretching beyond this limit is dangerous and it will harm more than benefit. Continuous practice and patience will make you perfect in asanas.

Sukhasana (easy pose)

Position:

- Take position with the legs straight in front of the body.
- Bend the right leg and place the foot under the left thigh.
- Bend the left leg and place the foot under the right thigh.
- Place the hands on knees. The arms should be relaxed and not held straight.
- Keep the head, neck and backbone upright and straight.
- Close the eyes and relax as long as you can.

Benefits:

This is the easiest and most comfortable pose in all the asanas. It facilitates mental and physical balance without causing strain or pain. It prepares you for more difficult asanas and pranayama practice at a later stage.

Note:

If you can sit in this asana for about an hour without doing any thing, it will enhance your concentration, memory. Just sit with closed eyes and observe the silence. Do not bother with the thoughts. Think what ever you like.

Vajrasana:

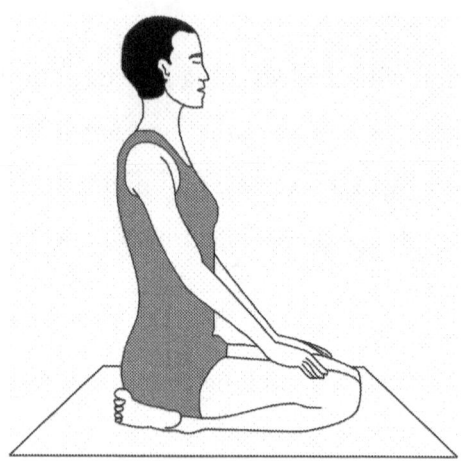

Position:

- Kneel on the floor.
- Bring the big toes together and separate the heels.
- Lower the buttocks onto the inside surface of the feet with the heels touching the sides of the hips.
- Place the hands on the knees, with palms down.
- The back and head should be straight but not tense.
- Avoid excess backward arching of the spine.
- Close the eyes, relax the arms and whole body.
- Breath normally and focus the attention on the flow of the air passing in and out of the nostrils.

Duration:

Practice vajrasana as much as possible, especially directly after meals, for at least 5 minutes, to enhance the digestive function. In cases of acute digestive disorder, sit in vajrasana and practice abdominal breathing for 100 breaths before and after food.

Benefits:

Vajrasana alters the flow of blood and nervous impulses in the pelvic region and strengthens the pelvic muscles. It is a preventive measure against hernia and it also helps to relieve piles. It increases the efficiency of the entire digestive system, relieving stomach ailments such as hyperacidity and peptic ulcer. It reduces the blood flow to the genitals and massages the nerve fibers which feed them. This is useful in the treatment of dilated testicles and hydrocele in men. It assists women in labor and helps alleviate menstrual disorder.

Vajrasana is a very important posture because the body becomes upright and straight with no effort. It is the best and easy meditation asana for people suffering from sciatica and sacral infections. It stimulates vajra nadi, activates prana in sushumna, and redirects sexual energy to the brain for spiritual purpose.

Note:

If there is pain in the thighs, the knees may be separated slightly while maintaining the posture. Beginners may find that their ankles ache after a short time in vajrasana. To remedy this, release the posture, sit with legs stretched forward and shake the feet vigorously one after the other until the stiffness disappears. Then resume the posture. A folded blanket or small cushion may be placed between the buttocks and the heels for added comfort.

Vajrasana is used by Muslims and Zen Buddhists as a position for their prayers and meditation. People, who cannot perform Padmasana or Siddhasana or who find them uncomfortable, may sit in vajrasana for meditation practice.

Shashankasana (pose of the moon):

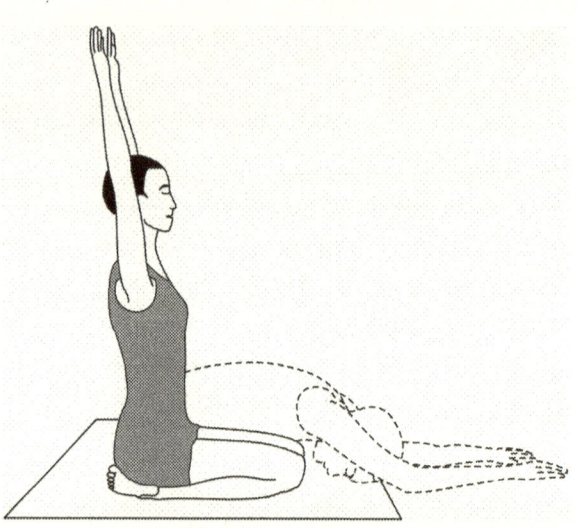

Position:

- Sit in vajrasana, placing the palms on the thighs just above the knees.

- Close the eyes and relax, keeping the spine and head straight.

- While inhaling, raise the arms above the head, keeping them straight and shoulder width apart.

- Exhale while bending the trunk forward from the hips, keeping the arms and head straight and in line with the trunk.

- At the end of the movement, the hands and forehead should rest on the floor in front of the knees.

- If possible, the arms and forehead should touch the floor at the same time.

- Bend the arms slightly so that they are fully relaxed, and let the elbows rest on the floor.

- Retain the breath for about 5 seconds in the final position.

- Then, simultaneously inhale and slowly raise the arms and trunk to the vertical position. Keep the arms head in line with the trunk. Breath out while lowering the arms to the knees.
- This is one round. Practice 3 to 5 rounds.

Position 2:

- In the final position of the above, bend both hands backward, placing besides the legs and palms facing upward.
- This gives extra pressure on chest and abdominal area.
- Stay in this position for a few seconds to few minutes.
- Return to the previous position.

Duration:

Beginners should slowly increase the length of time in the final position until they are able to hold it comfortably for at least 3 minutes. Those who wish to calm anger and frayed nerves should further increase the time upto 10 minutes, breathing normally.

Warning:

Not to be performed by people with very high blood pressure, slipped disc or those who suffer from vertigo.

Benefits:

This asana stretches the back muscles and separates the individual vertebrae from one another, releasing pressure on discs. Often nerve connections emanating from the spinal cord are squeezed by these discs, giving rise to various forms of backache. This posture helps to relieve this problem and encourages the discs to resume their correct position.

It also regulates the functioning of the adrenal glands. It tones the pelvic muscles and the sciatic nerves and is beneficial to women who have an underdeveloped pelvis. It helps to alleviate disorders of both the male and female reproductive organs.

Regular practice relieves constipation. When practiced with Ujjayi pranayama in the final position, it helps to eliminate anger and rage, and is very cooling for the brain.

Gomukhasana (Cow's face pose)

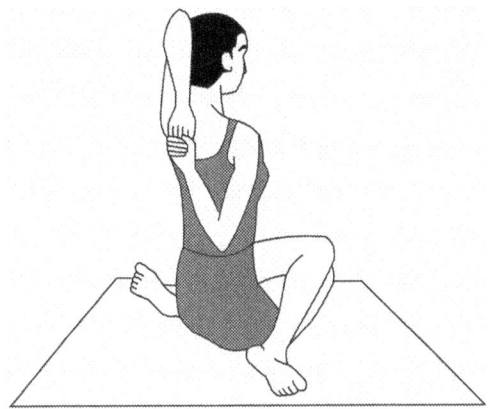

Position:

- Sit in dhyana veerasana so that the right knee is directly above the left knee as shown in the picture.
- Place the left arm behind the back and the right arm over the right shoulder.
- The back of the hand should lie in contact with the spine while the palm of the right hand rests against the spine.
- Try to clasp the fingers of both hands behind the back.
- Bring the raised elbow behind the head so that the head presses against the inside of the raised arm.
- If you feel difficulties in the above process, then simply put the hands on the knees.
- The spine should be erect and the head back. Close the eyes.
- Stay in this position for 2 to 3 minutes.
- Unclasp the hands, straighten the legs and repeat, with the left knee uppermost and the left arm over the left shoulder.
- Breath normally during this asana.

Benefits:

Gomukhasana is an excellent asana for inducting relaxation. If practiced for 10 minutes or more, it will alleviate tiredness, tension and anxiety. It stimulates the kidneys and alleviates mature, onset diabetes. It relieves backache, sciatica, rheumatism, and general stiffness in the shoulders and the neck, and improves posture by opening the chest area. It alleviates cramp in the legs and makes the leg muscles supple.

Wakrasana (spinal twist):

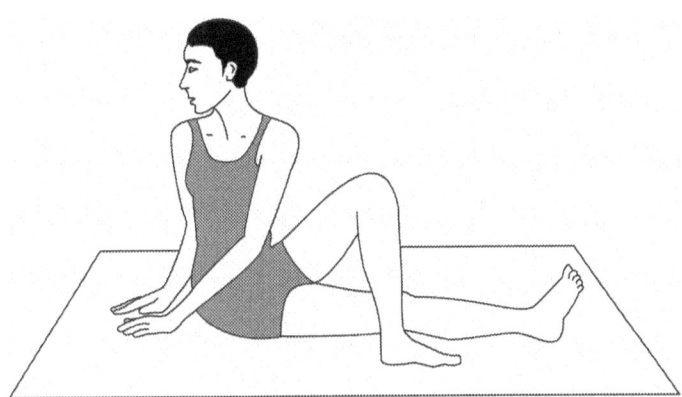

Position:

- Sit with the legs outstretched.
- Turn the trunk slightly to the right and place the right hand behind the body, close to the left buttock.
- Place the left hand behind to the side of the right buttock, as close as possible to the right hand.
- Bend the left knee and place the foot outside the right knee.
- Turn the head and body to the right as comfortable as possible.
- Use the arms as support while keeping the spine upright and straight.
- Look back over the right shoulder and relax.
- Stay in this position for a few seconds.
- Return to the starting position and repeat on left side.
- Practice up to 4 rounds.

Breathing:

Inhale before twisting. Retain the breath inside while twisting. Exhale while re-centering.

Benefits:

This asana stretches the spine, loosening the vertebrae and toning the nerves. It alleviates backache, neck pain, and mild form of sciatica. It is a good asana for beginners.

Padmasana (lotus pose)

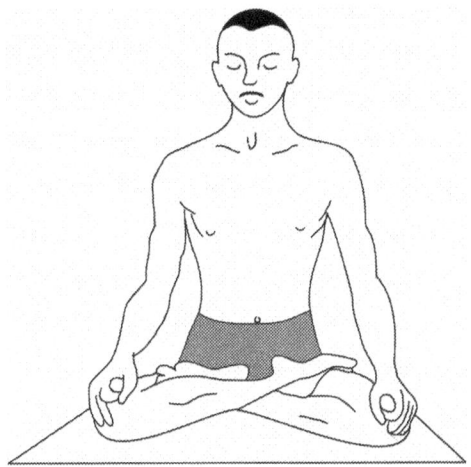

Position:

- Sit with the legs straight in front of the body.
- Slowly and carefully bend one leg and place the foot on the top of the opposite thigh.
- The sole should face upward and the heels should be close to the pubic bone.
- When this feels comfortable, bend the other leg and place the foot on top of the opposite thigh.
- Both knees should, ideally, touch the ground in the final position.
- The head and spine should be held upright and the shoulders relaxed.
- Place the hands on the knees in chin mudra as shown in the picture.
- Close the eyes and relax the whole body.

- Observe the total posture of the body. Make the necessary adjustment by moving forward or backward until balance and alignment are experienced.

- If not possible with both legs, in the beginning, try with only one leg (called half Padmasana).

Benefits:

Padmasana allows the body to be held completely steady for long periods of time. It holds the trunk and head like a pillar, with the legs as the firm foundation. As the body is steadied, the mind becomes calm very fast.

This posture applies pressure to the lower spine which has a relaxing effect on the nervous system. The breath becomes slow, muscular tension is decreased and blood pressure is reduced.

Yogamudrasana (Psychic union pose)

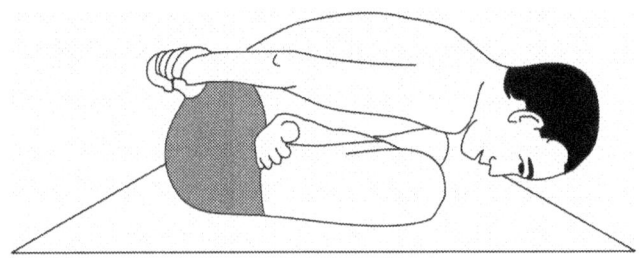

Position:

- Sit in Padmasana and close eyes. In the beginning, you can start with half Padmasana.
- Relax the body and breath normally for a few seconds.
- Hold one wrist behind the back with the other hand as shown in the picture.
- Inhale deeply. While exhaling, bend forward, keeping the spine straight.
- Bring the forehead to the floor or as close to the floor as possible.
- Relax the whole body, breath slowly and deeply. Be aware of the pressure of the heels on the abdomen.
- Stay in the position as far as you can.
- Slowly return to the final position.
- Repeat the pose with the legs crossed the other way.

Breathing:

Inhale slowly and deeply in the starting position. Exhale while bending forward. Breath deeply and slowly in the final position. Inhale while returning to the starting pose.

Titali (butterfly pose):

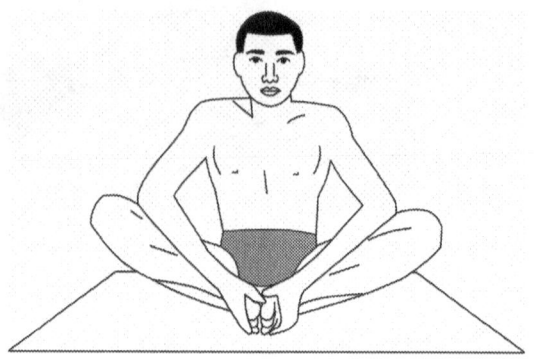

Position 1:

- Sit in sukhasana.

- Bend the knees and bring the soles of the feet together.

- Keep the heels as close to the body as possible.

- Fully relax the inner thigh muscles.

- Clasp the feet with both hands.

- Gently bounce the knees up and down, using the elbows as levers to press the legs down.

- Try to touch the knees to the ground on downward stroke. Do not use any force.

- Practice 25 to 40 ups and down.

Position 2:

- Place the hands on the knees.

- Using the palms, gently push the knees down towards the floor, allowing them to spring up again.

- Do not use the force for this movement.
- Straighten the legs and relax the whole body.

Benefits:

The inner thigh muscles hold a lot of tension, which is relieved by these asanas. They also remove tiredness caused by long hours of standing and walking.

Pada Hastasana (forward bending Pose)

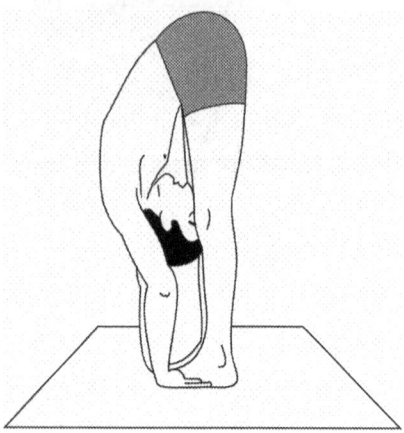

Position:

- Stand with the spine erect, feet together and hands beside the body. Relax for a few seconds.

- Slowly bend forward, first bending the head, taking the chin towards the chest, then bending the upper trunk, relaxing the shoulders forward and letting the arms go limp.

- Do not strain or force the body. In the beginning, a complete bend, as shown in the picture, is not possible. Try slowly and steadily over a period of time to reach the toes of the feet.

Final Position

- Bring the palms to the floor beside the feet.

- If this is not possible, bring the fingertips as near to the floor as possible.

- In the final position, the body is bent forward with the knees straight and the forehead touching the knees.

- Slowly return to the final position in the reverse order. Relax the body in the upright position and feel the pain in the leg and the back.

- Repeat the whole process again.

Breathing:

Inhale in the starting position. Exhale while bending forward. Breath slowly and deeply in the final position.

Duration:

Practice up to 4 or 5 rounds, gradually increasing the time for which the posture is held and decreasing the numbers of rounds, or practice one round for 3 to 4 minutes.

Benefits:

This asana massages and tones the digestive organs, alleviate constipation and indigestion. All the spinal nerves are stimulated and toned. Inverting the trunk increases the blood flow to the brain and improves circulation to the pituitary and thyroids glands. Other benefits are increased vitality, improved metabolism, increased concentration and the removal of nasal and throat diseases. It also helps to reduce excess weight.

Paschimottanasana (back stretching pose)

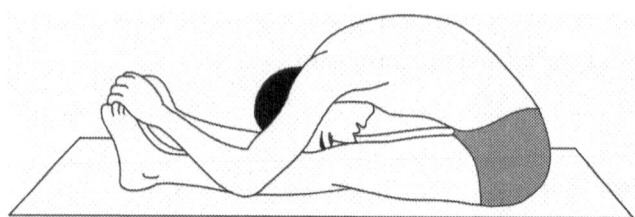

Position:

- Sit on the floor with legs outstretched, feet together and hands on the knees.

- Relax the whole body for a few seconds.

- Slowly bend forward from hips and try to hold the big toes with fingers and thumbs.

- If this is not possible, then hold any part of the legs.

- Move slowly without forcing or jerking.

- Hold the position for a few seconds. Relax the back and the leg muscles, allowing them to stretch gently.

- Try to touch the knees with the forehead. Do not strain and force.

- Hold the position as long as comfortable.

- Slowly return to the original position.

Breathing:

Inhale in the starting position. Exhale slowly while bending forward. Breath slowly and deeply in the final position. Inhale while returning to the starting position.

Benefits:

This asana stretches the hamstring muscles and increase flexibility in the hip joints. It tones and massages the entire abdominal and pelvic region, including the liver, pancreas, spleen, kidneys and adrenal glands. It removes excess weight in this area.

Trikonasana (Triangle Pose):

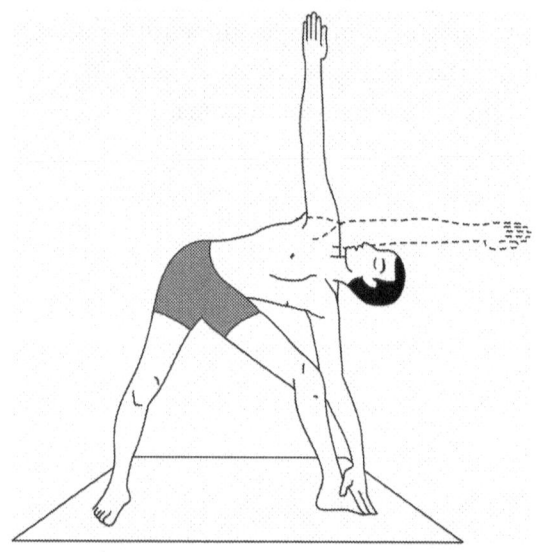

Position 1:

- Stand erect with the feet about a meter apart.
- Turn the right foot to the right side.
- Stretch the arms sideways and raise them to shoulders level so that they are in one straight horizontal line.
- Bend to the right, but not forward.
- Simultaneously bend the right knee slightly.
- Place the right hand on the right foot, keeping the two arms in line with each other as shown in the picture.
- Look up at the left hand in the final position.
- Return to the upright position, with the arms in a straight line.
- Repeat on the opposite side.
- Practice 5 rounds.

Position 2:

- Repeat the process as in the above position 1.
- Keep the upper arm over the ear until it is parallel to the floor, with the palm facing down as shown in the picture.
- Look up at the left hand.
- Do not bend forward but keep the body in one vertical plane.
- Repeat on the left side.

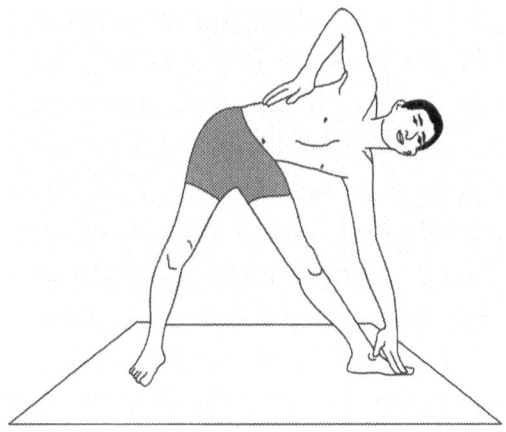

Position 3:

- Stand with the feet one meter apart.
- Place the palms of the hands on each side of the waist, with the fingers pointing downward.
- Breathing out, slowly bend to the right from the hips while sliding the right hand down along the outside of the right thigh as far as possible.
- Do not strain and do not bend to get to final position.
- Hold there for a few seconds, holding the breath.
- Repeat on the left side.

- Practice 4 to 5 rounds.

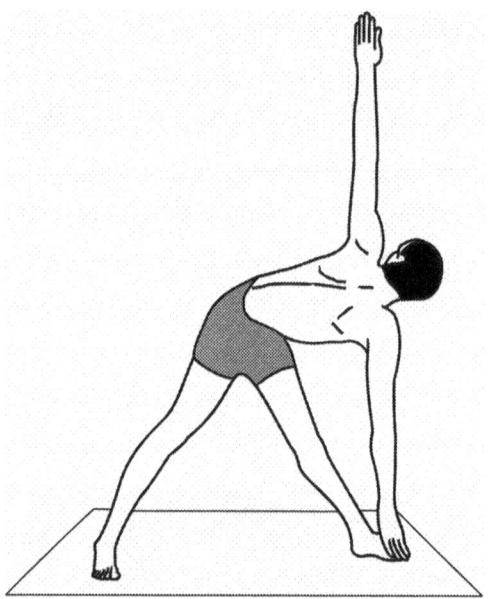

Position 4:

- While breathing in, raise the arms sideways to shoulder level.
- While breathing out, bend forward. Twist the trunk to the left, bringing the right hand to the left foot.
- The left arm should be outstretched vertically as shown in picture.
- Look up at the left hand.
- Hold the breath, feel the twist and stretch of the back.
- Repeat on the opposite side.
- Practice 5 rounds.

Benefits:

After a few weeks of practice of all these four positions, the entire body will be toned. It stimulates the nervous system. It improves digestion, stimulating appetite, activating intestinal peristalsis and alleviating constipation. Regular practice will help to reduce the waistline fat.

Important Note:

Increasing the distance between the feet gives a more powerful stretch to the rarely used inner thigh muscles and the top of the thighs.

Tadasana (Palm Tree pose):

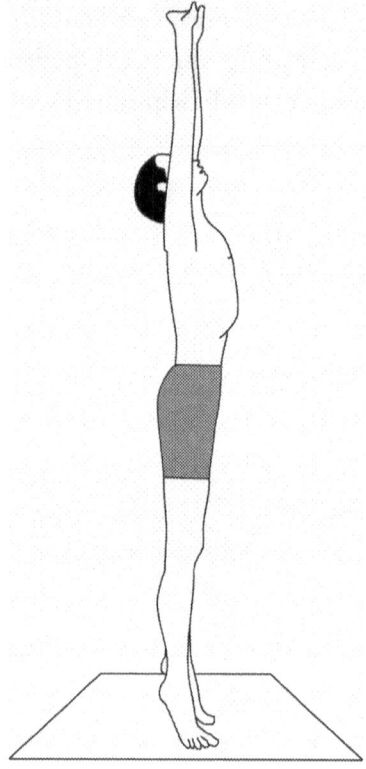

Position:

- Stand with the feet about 10 cm apart and arms by the sides.
- Raise the arms over the head in the vertical line of the body.
- Keep the palms of the hands facing inside, and about 10 cm apart.
- Inhale and stretch the arms, shoulders and chest upward. Raise the heels coming up onto the toes.
- Stretch the whole body from top to bottom, without losing balance or moving the feet.

- Hold the breath and the position for a few seconds.

- Lower the heels while breathing out and bring the hands to the sides.

- Relax for a few seconds and perform the next round. Practice 3 to 5 rounds.

Benefits:

This asana develops physical and mental balance. The entire spine is stretched and loosened, helping to clear up congestion of the spinal nerves at the points where they emerge from the spinal column. Tadasana stretches the rectus abdominal muscles and the intestines, and is useful during the first six months of pregnancy in order to keep the abdominal muscles and nerves toned.

Bhujangasana (cobra pose)

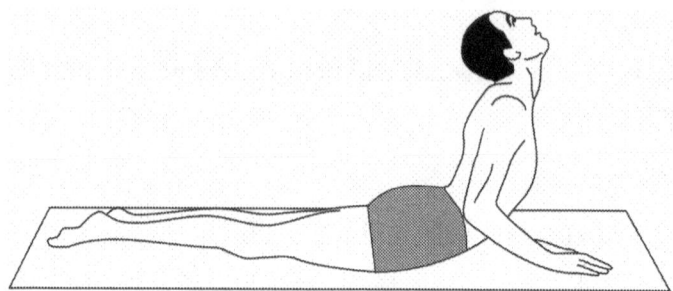

Position:

- Lie flat on the stomach with legs straight, feet together and the soles of the feet uppermost as shown in picture.
- Place the palms of the hands flat on the floor, below and slightly to the side of the shoulders.
- The fingers should be together and pointing forward.
- The arms should be positioned so that the elbows point backward and are close to the sides of the body.
- Rest the forehead on the floor and close the eyes.
- Relax the body.
- Slowly raise the head, neck and shoulders. Straightening the elbows, raise the trunk as high as possible. Use the back muscles more than the arm muscles.
- Be aware of using the back muscles first while starting to raise the trunk. Then use the arm muscles to raise the trunk further and arch the back.
- Gently tilt the head backward, so that the chin points forward and the back of the neck is compressed.
- Hold the final position for few seconds to one minute.

- Slowly bring the head forward, release the upper back by bending the arms, lower the navel, chest, shoulders and finally the forehead to the floor.

- Relax the whole body, specially the lower back muscles. This is one round. Practice up to 5 rounds.

Breathing:

Breathing in while raising the trunk. Breath normally while in final position and breathing out while lowering the trunk.

Benefits:

This asana is very good to relocate the slipped disc, remove backache and keep the backbone healthy and straight. A stiff spine interferes with all nervous impulses sent from the brain to the body and vice versa. By arching the spine, improving circulation in the back region and toning the nerves, resulting in better communication between the brain and body. It stimulates the appetite, alleviates constipation and is beneficial for all the abdominal organs, especially the liver and kidneys.

Naukasana (boat pose)

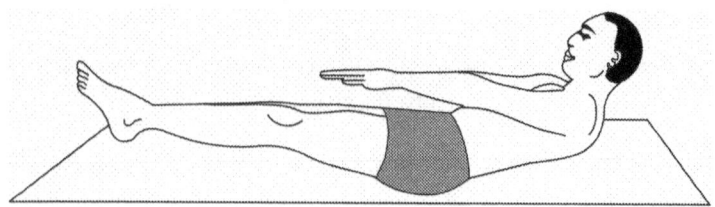

Position:

- Lie on the floor with face up ward. Hands besides the body with palms down.

- Breath in deeply. While holding the breath, raise the legs, arms and shoulders, head and trunk off the ground as shown in the picture.

- The shoulders and feet should be raised to around 6" from the floor.

- Balance the body on the buttocks and keep the spine straight.

- The arms should be held at the same level and in the line with the toes. The hands should be open with the palms down.

- Look towards the toes. Eyes should remain open during asana.

- Remain in final position for few seconds and return to the beginning pose with great care.

- Close the eyes and relax the body.

Breathing:

Inhale while raising the body and exhale while lowering the body. Retain the breath while in final position.

Benefits:

This asana helps to improve the muscular, digestive, blood circulation, nervous and hormonal systems, tones all the organs and removes laziness. It is best to perform before shavasana in order to attain a deeper state of relaxation.

Dhanurasana (Bow Pose)

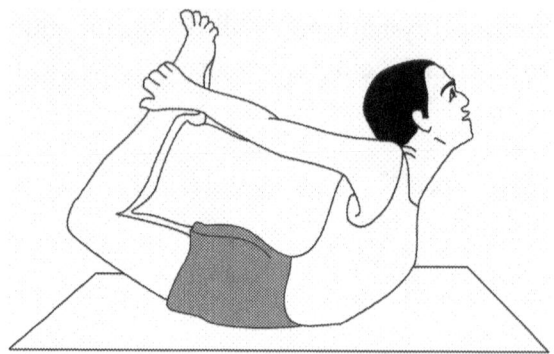

Position:

- Lie flat on the stomach, with the legs and feet together and the arms and hands beside the body.

- Bend the knees and bring the heels close to the buttocks.

- Clasp the hand around the ankles and place the chin on the floor.

- Arch the back, lifting the thighs, chest and head together as shown in the picture.

- Keep the arms straight.

- The only muscular contraction is in the legs; the back and the arms remain relaxed.

- Release the position and relax until the breath returns to normal.

Benefits:

The entire alimentary canal is reconditioned by this asana. The liver, abdominal organs and muscles are massaged. The pancreas and adrenal glands are toned. The kidneys are massaged and excess weight is reduced around the abdominal area.

This leads to improved functioning of the digestive, eliminative and reproductive organs, and helps to remove the gastrointestinal disorders, chronic constipation and sluggishness of the liver.

Dhanurasana is useful for relieving various chest ailments, including asthma, and freeing nervous energy in the cervical and thoracic sympathetic nerves, eventually improving the respiration.

Shalabhasana (locust pose)

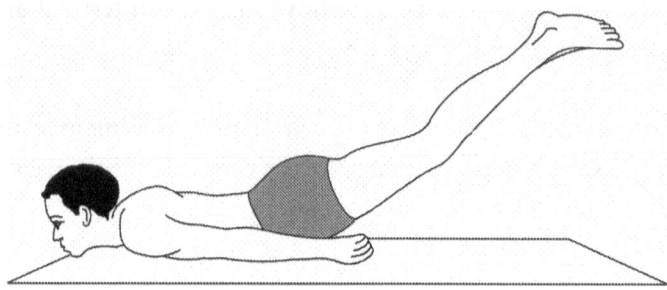

Position:

- Lie on the stomach with the legs and feet together and the soles of the feet uppermost.

- The arms may be placed either under the body or by the sides, with the palms downward.

- Stretch the chin slightly forward and rest it on the floor throughout the practice of this asana.

- Close the eyes and relax the body.

- Slowly raise the legs as high as possible, keeping them straight and together.

- The elevation of the legs is produced by applying pressure with the arms against the floor.

- Remain in final position as long as possible and comfortable.

- Slowly lower the legs to the floor.

- Relax the whole body and remain in base position for one minute.

Breathing:

Inhale long breath in beginning position. Hold the breath while raising the legs and during the final position. Exhale while lowering the legs to the floor.

Benefits:

This asana strengthens the lower back and pelvic organs, massages the nervous system, providing relief to backache, slipped disc. It improves the efficiency of the liver and other abdominal organs, alleviate diseases of the stomach and bowels, and stimulate the appetite.

Makarasana (crocodile pose)

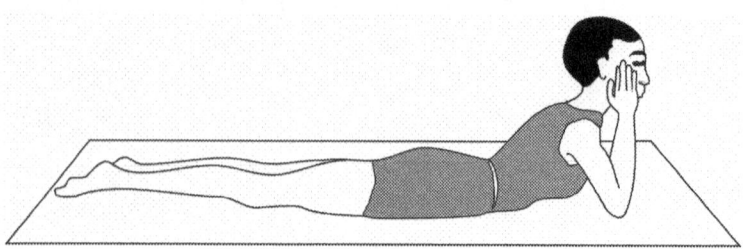

Position;

- Lie flat on the stomach.

- Raise the head and the shoulders and rest the chin in the palms of the hands with the elbows on the floor.

- Keep the elbows together. Separate the elbows slightly to relieve pressure on the neck.

- Experience the strain at the neck when the elbows are too far from each other. The strain will be experienced at the lower back when they close together.

- Adjust the elbows so that the whole spine is equally relaxed.

- While resting, move the eyes up and down, or rotate the eye balls from right to left and left to right.

- Relax and close the eyes.

Benefits:

This asana should be practiced for quiet a long time to get its benefits. It is very helpful to people suffering from slipped disc, lower back pain or any other spinal disorder. This asana is very good for relaxation after other asana practice.

Shavasana (corpse pose)

Position:

- Lie flat on the back with the arms about 15 cm away from the body, palms facing upward.
- Let the fingers curl up slightly.
- Move the feet slightly apart to a comfortable position and close the eyes.
- The head and spine should be in a straight line.
- Relax the whole body and stop all physical movements.
- Become aware of the natural breath and allow it to become rhythmic.

Duration:

Practice this asana as and when the time is available. The longer is the better, although two minutes are sufficient between two asana practices.

Benefits:

This asana relaxes the whole psycho—physiological system. It should ideally be practiced before sleep; before, during and after asana practice. When you feel physically and mentally tired, this asana is very good to revitalize the body. It develops body awareness. This is the best asana to get relaxed and it is very easy to do.

Sirshasana (headstand pose):

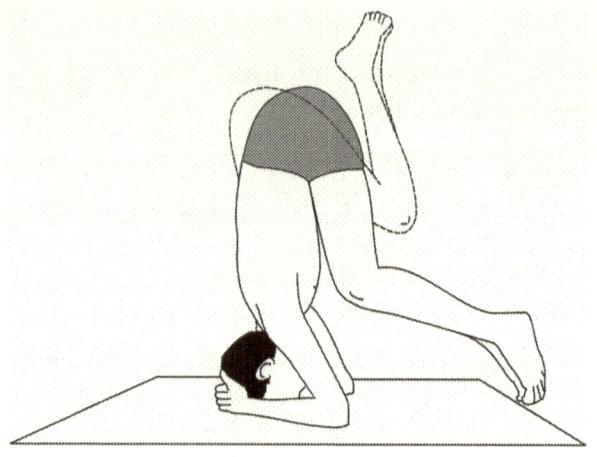

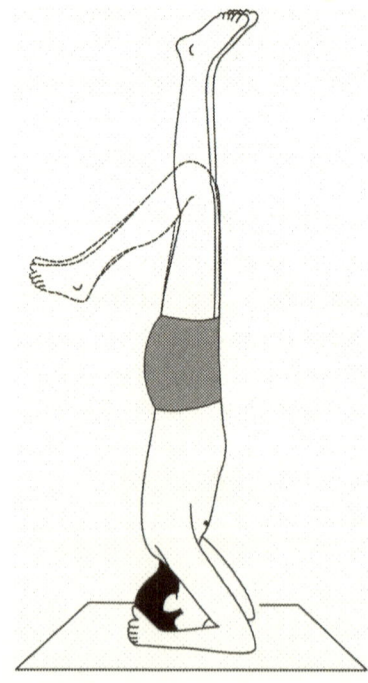

Position: Initially take the support of a wall for balance.

Stage 1):

- Sit in Vajrasana, close the eyes and relax the whole body.

- After a few minutes, open the eyes, bend forward and place the forearms on a folded blanket or cushion, with fingers interlocked and the elbows in front of the knees.

- Place the crown of the head between the interlocked fingers on the blanket. Wrap the hands around the head to make a firm support so that it cannot roll backward when pressure is applied.

Stage 2):

- Lift the knees and buttocks off the floor and straighten the legs up in the air. Transfer the weight onto the head and arms simultaneously.

Stage 3):

- The whole body should be in one straight line with the feet relaxed. Balance the body with the support of the wall. Close the eyes and balance the body, relaxing in the final position for as long as is comfortable.

- Return to the starting position. Slowly bend the knees and lower the body with control in the reverse order until the toes touch the floor. Remain with the head on the ground in the kneeling position for a short time, and then slowly return to the vajrasana position.

Breathing:

Inhale at the end of the stage 1. Hold the breath during the lifting of the body to the last position. Breath normally during the asanas.

Duration:

Initially start this asana for 30 to 60 seconds. Slowly add 30 more seconds and go for up to 5 minutes. This duration is enough for good health.

Benefits:

This asana is very powerful for awakening Sahastra Chakra and, therefore, it is considered the greatest of all the asanas.

Sirshasana increases the blood flow to the brain and the pituitary gland, revitalizing the entire body and mind. It relieves anxiety and other psychological disturbances which form the root cause of many disorders. It is therefore recommended for the prevention of asthma, hey fever, diabetes and menopausal imbalance. Importantly, it increases the memory power, thus reducing the chance of the occurring of the Alzheimer disease.

This asana reverse the effect of gravity on the spine. Strain on the back is thus alleviated and the reversed flow of blood in the legs and visceral regions aids the tissue regeneration. The weight of the abdominal organs on the diaphragm encourages deep exhalation so that larger amounts of carbon dioxide, toxins and bacteria are removed from the lungs.

Note:

In the final position, most of the weight of the body is sustained by the top of the head, arms being used to maintain balance only. Beginners, however, may use the arms as support until the neck is strong enough to bear the full weight of the body.

If the practitioner should have a fall during the practice, the body should be as relaxed as possible. If the fall is forward, try to fold the knees into the chest so that the impact on the floor is sustained by the feet.

Sarvangasana (shoulder stand pose):

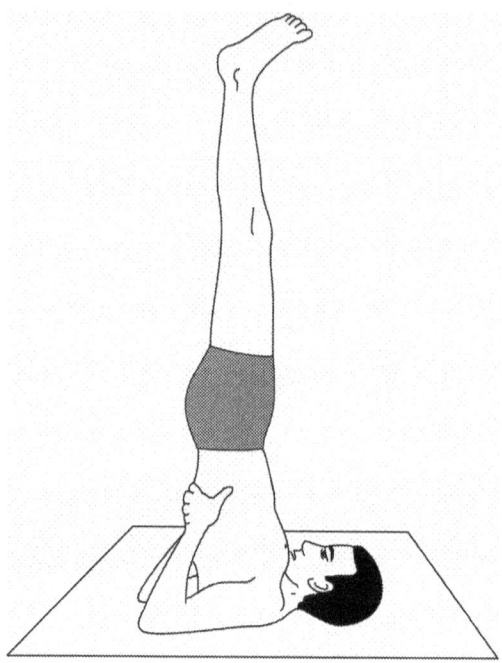

Position:

- Lie on the back on a folded blanket. Check that the head and spine are aligned and that the legs are straight, with the feet together.

- Place the hands beside the body with the palms facing down.

- Relax the entire body and mind.

- With the support of the arms, slowly raise the legs to the vertical position, keeping them straight.

- When the legs are vertical, press the arms and hands down on the floor. Slowly and smoothly roll the buttocks and spine off the floor, raising the trunk to a vertical position.

- Turn the palms of the hands upward, bend the elbows and place the hands behind the ribcage, slightly away from the spine, to support the back. The elbows should be about shoulder width apart.

- Gently push the chest forward so that it presses firmly against the chin.

- In the final position, the legs are vertically together and in a straight line with the trunk. The body is supported by the shoulders, the back of the neck and the back of the head. The arms provide stability, the chest rests against the chin and the feet are relaxed.

- Close the eyes. Relax the whole body and stay in the position as long as comfortable.

- To return to the starting position, bring the legs forward until the feet are above and behind the back of the head. Keep the legs straight.

- Slowly release the position of the hands and place the arms on the floor beside the body, with palms down.

- Gradually lower each vertebrae of the spine to the floor, followed by the buttocks, so that the legs resume their initial vertical position.

- Lower the legs to the floor slowly, keeping the knees straight.

- Perform this action without using the arms for support. The body should contact the floor slowly and gently.

- Relax in shavasana until respiration and heart beats return to normal.

Breathing:

Inhale in the starting position. Hold the breath inside while assuming the final pose. Practice slow, deep abdominal breathing in the final pose. Hold the breath inside while lowering the body to the floor.

Duration:

Beginners should hold the final position for a few seconds only, gradually increasing to a maximum of 3 to 5 minutes for general health. This asana should be performed only once during the session.

Benefits:

By pressing the chest against the chin, this asana stimulates the thyroid gland, balancing the circulatory, digestive, reproductive, nervous and endocrine systems. Together with the enriched blood flow to the brain, it also tranquillizes the mind, relieves mental and emotional stress, fear and headache. This also helps clear psychological disturbances. The thymus gland is also stimulated, boosting the immune system.

Sarvangasana releases the normal gravitational pressure from the anal muscles, relieving hemorrhoids. It tones the legs, abdomen and reproductive organs, draining stagnant blood and fluid, and increasing circulation to these areas.

This asana is used in yoga therapy for the treatment of asthma, diabetes, colitis, thyroid disorder, impotence, hydrocele, prolapse, menopause menstrual disorders and leucorrhoea. Regular practice helps to prevent cough, cold and flu.

Aerobic exercise: Fit for Hit

Besides the asanas, the body needs some kind of aerobic exercise. The best way to slow the ageing process and ensure good health is a combination of exercise and proper nutrition. Regular exercise improves digestion, calumniation, energy levels, lowers cholesterol, elevates your mood and reduces anxiety and depression.

Exercise can be recreational as well as therapeutic. Brisk walking or slow jogging is the best aerobic exercise because you do not need anybody for company. Moreover, there is no cost at all. The important thing to remember is that you should indulge in those exercises which you are most comfortable with.

Certain games are also good aerobic exercises. Badminton, lawn tennis, volleyball, basketball or any other sports you love to play. During aerobic exercise, heart beats rapidly and breathing becomes very rapid.

Fitness is a combination of mental and physical health and both are correlated—if you are happy, it reflects in your health, skin and hair. It also means emotional and spiritual wee-being. Sheer determination and hard work are very important to be in shape. It is important to be physically active to be healthy.

7

Breathing (Pranayama): Source of Life

Most of the people use only a fraction of their lung capacity for breathing during their life time. They breath shallowly, barely expanding the ribcage. Their shoulders are hunched; they have painful tension in the upper part of the back and neck, and they suffer from lack of oxygen. They should learn the full Yogic breathing.

Observe your breathing when you are getting anxious about something; your breath is blocked due to an involuntary contraction in the chest. The simple truth is that "Deeper the anxiety, longer the blockade". Imagine the situation when you are getting ready for office in the morning. You are unable to locate your keys. You ask your spouse to help you find the same. Your spouse is busy and asks you to wait. You burst into a temper. At that moment you will observe that your inhalation is held up, depriving you of the vitality of fresh air due to the contraction of the chest and the diaphragm.

This deficiency is the result of shallow and irregular breathing. We never take breathing seriously but always neglect it. Therefore we keep breathing shallow and short. There is hardly any occasion when we have breathed deeply by fully expanding the abdomen and the chest from bottom to apex. It is therefore not surprising that most of the people suffer from over-reaction, stress and lack of concentration.

Deep breathing makes you a good listener, too. You will be able to understand the viewpoint of others and to deal with problems effectively. It enhances mental stability and the ability to concentrate. As you learn how to breath deeply, compulsive arousal of emotions get diluted and the energy held by them is released for better and creative performance.

Whenever you are confronted with an inconvenient situation, take care to start breathing deeply before tackling the problems such as facing an interview for a job, giving a presentation at a meeting or in public. After a few trials, you will overcome any deficiency. Ideas, which caused stress earlier, will no longer do so, and you can lead a stable and delightful life.

One way to regulate deep breathing is to practice pranayama regularly.

Different Types of Breathing

Clavicular breathing is the most shallow and the worst possible type. The shoulders and collarbones are raised while the abdomen is contracted during inhalation. Maximum effort is made, but a minimum amount of air is obtained.

Thoracic breathing is done with the rib muscles expanding the rib cage, and is the second type of incomplete breathing.

Deep abdominal breathing is the best, because it brings air into the lowest and the largest part of the lungs. Breathing should be slow and deep, and proper use should be made of the diaphragm.

Actually, none of these types are complete. A full Yogic breath combines all these three types, beginning with a deep breath and continuing the inhalation through the intercostals and clavicular areas.

Learning the Abdominal Breathing

To get the feel of proper diaphragmatic breathing, wear loose clothing and lie on the back. Place the hand on the upper abdomen, where the diaphragm is located. Breath in and out slowly. The abdomen should expand outward as you inhale and contract as you exhale. Try to get the feeling of this motion.

Learning the Full Yogic Breathing

Once you feel proficient in the practice of the abdominal breathing, you will be ready to learn the Full Yogic Breathing. Breath in slowly; expand the abdomen, then the ribcage, and finally the upper portion of the lungs. Then, breath out in the same manner, letting the abdomen cave in as you exhale. This is the complete Yogic breath.

Once you learn complete yogic breathing, you are now ready to practice the pranayama. Pranayama should be performed in sukhasana or vajrasana, holding the chest, throat, and head erect. The best time to do the pranayama is early morning when the outside atmosphere is calm and quiet. The air is fresh and the mind is free from any stress.

After practicing for about a week, you can experience the delight of deep breathing-as a parent, as marketing executive, as an interviewer or as any other professional. Next time, before meeting a client, have a session of deep breathing for five minutes. You will be astonished at your performance. You will discover that you are possessed with a new found energy and elegance; the way you interact with your clients undergoes a perceptible change.

Pranayama

By far, the most important thing about good breathing is the Prana, or the subtle energy of the vital breath. Control of the Prana leads to the control of the mind. Breathing exercises are called Pranayama, which means controlling the Prana. The word pranayama is comprised of two roots: prana and ayama.

Prana means vital energy or force of life. It is more subtle than air or oxygen. Therefore, pranayama should not be considered as a mere breathing exercise. Pranayama utilizes breathing to influence the flow of prana in the nadis or energy channels.

The word yama means control and it is used to denote various rules or codes of conduct during practicing pranayama.

Four aspects of pranayama:

- Inhalation
- Exhalation
- Internal breath retention
- External breath retention

The different practices of pranayama use various techniques, which utilize these four aspects of breathing. The most important part of pranayama is actually breath retention.

Breathing is so simple and obvious that we often take it for granted, ignoring the power it has to affect body, mind and spirit. With each inhale, we bring oxygen into the body and spark the transformation of nutrients into fuel. Each exhale purges the body of carbon dioxide, toxic waste. Breathing also affects our state of mind. It can make us excited or calm, tense or relaxed. It can make our thinking confused or clear. What is more, in the yogic tradition, air is the primary source of prana or life force, a psycho-physio-spiritual force that permeates the universe.

Pranayama is loosely translated as prana or breath control. The ancient yogis developed many breathing techniques to maximize the benefits of prana. Pranayama is used in yoga as a separate practice to help clear and cleanse the body and mind. It is also used in preparation for meditation, and in asanas, the practice of postures, to help maximize the benefits of the practice, and to focus on the mind.

Pranayama is the only way through which we can clean our internal organs. When we take a bath, we clean only the external body but we can not see our internal organs on which toxins are accumulated. If we breath rhythmically and deeply, our all internal organs including many cells and tissues get fresh oxygen; the whole internal system becomes rejuvenated and we become disease free.

Below are several of the most commonly used forms of pranayama.

1. Ujjayi Pranayama

2. Dirgha Pranayama

3. Anulom—Viloma Pranayama

4. Brahmari Pranayama

5. Bhastrika Pranayama

6. Seetkari Pranayama

1) Ujjayi Pranayama

Ujjayi is often called the "sounding" breath or "ocean sounding" breath, somewhat irreverently called as the "Darth Vader" breath. It involves constricting the back of the throat while breathing to create an "ah" sound—thus the names for various types of sounding.

Benefits: Focuses the mind; Increases mindfulness; Generates internal heat.

How to do it:

- Take a comfortable seated position, with your spine erect; or, lie down on your back. Begin taking long, slow, and deep breaths through the nostrils.

- Allow the breath to be gentle and relaxed as you slightly contract the back of your throat creating a steady hissing sound as you breath in and out. The sound need not be forced, but it should be loud enough so that if someone came close to you they would hear it.

- Lengthen the inhalation and the exhalation as much as possible without creating tension anywhere in your body, and allow the sound of the breath to be continuous and smooth.

To help create the proper "ah" sound, hold your hand up to your mouth and exhale as if trying to fog a mirror. Inhale the same way. Notice how you constrict the back of the throat to create the fog effect. Now close your mouth and do the same thing while breathing through the nose.

When to do it:

During asana practice, before meditation, or at anytime you want to concentrate.

2) Dirgha Pranayama

Known as the "complete" or "three-part" breath, dirgha pranayama teaches how to fill the three chambers of the lungs, beginning with the lower lungs, and then moving up through the thoracic region and into the clavicular region.

Benefits:

Promotes proper diaphragmatic breathing, relaxes the mind and the body, oxygenates the blood and purges the lungs of residual carbon dioxide.

How to do it

Sit with your spine erect, or lie down on your back. Begin taking long, slow, and deep breaths through the nostrils.

As you inhale, allow the belly to fill with air, drawing air deep into the lower lungs. As you exhale, allow the belly to deflate like a balloon. Repeat several times, keeping the breath smooth and relaxed, and never straining. Repeat several times.

Breath into your belly as in Step #1, but also expand the mid-chest region by allowing the rib cage to open outward to the sides. Exhale and repeat several times.

Follow steps #1 and #2 and continue inhaling by opening the clavicular region or the upper chest. Exhale and repeat.

Combine all the three steps of breathing (as told in the beginning of this chapter) into one continuous or complete flow.

3) Anulom-Viloma Pranayama:

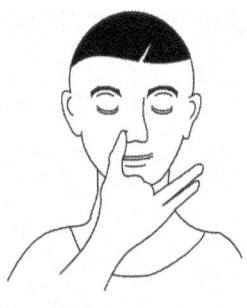

Anulom—Viloma or Nadi Shodhana, or the sweet breath, is a simple form of alternate nostril breathing suitable for the beginners. Nadi means a channel. It refers to the energy-pathways through which prana flows. Shodhana means cleansing—so Nadi Shodhana means channel cleaning.

How to do it:

- Hold your right hand up and curl your index and middle fingers toward your palm.
- Place your thumb next to your right nostril and your ring finger and pinky to your left.
- Close the left nostril by pressing gently against it with your ring finger and pinky, and inhale through the right nostril.
- The breath should be slow, steady and full.
- Now close the right nostril by pressing gently against it with your thumb, and open your left nostril by relaxing your ring finger and pinky and exhale fully with a slow and steady breath.
- Inhale through the left nostril, close it, and then exhale through the right nostril.
- That is one complete round of Nadi Shodhana

- Inhale through the right nostril, Exhale through the left, Inhale through the left, Exhale through the right.

- Begin with 5-10 rounds and add more as you feel ready. Remember to keep your breathing slow, easy and full.

When to do it:

Just at anytime and anywhere you want. Try it as a mental warm-up before meditation to help calm the mind and put you in a pleasing mood. You can also do it as part of your centering before beginning an asana or posture routine. Also try it at times throughout the day.

Benefits:

Calms the mind, soothes anxiety and stress, balances left and right hemispheres, and promotes clear thinking. Nadi Shodhana helps control stress and anxiety. If you start to feel stressed out, 10 or so rounds will help you calm down. It also helps soothe anxiety caused by flying and other fearful or stressful situations.

4) Brahmari Pranayama (humming bee breath):

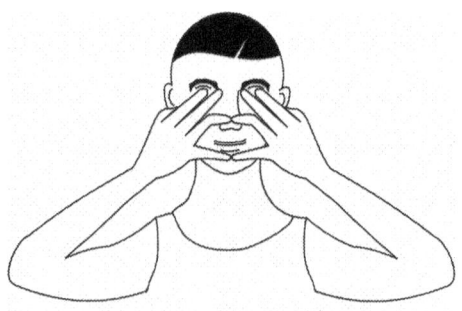

How to do it:

- Take a comfortable meditation posture. The spinal chord should be erect, the head straight and the hands resting on the knees.
- Close the eyes and relax the whole body for a few seconds.
- The lips should remain gently closed with the teeth slightly separated throughout the practice. This allows the sound vibration to be heard and felt more distinctly in the brain.
- Make sure the jaws are relaxed.
- Place the fingers as shown in the picture.
- Do not press a finger on a nostril too firmly.
- Bring total awareness to the centre of the head and keep the body absolutely still.
- Breath in through the nose slowly and deeply.
- Exhale slowly while making a deep, steady humming sound likes that of a black bee.
- The humming sound should be smooth, even and continuous for the duration of exhalation.
- At the end of exhalation, breath in deeply and repeat for 5 rounds.

Benefits:

Brahmari pranayama relieves stress and cerebral tension, alleviating anger, anxiety and insomnia. It reduces blood pressure and speeds up the healing of the body tissue; and it may be practiced after operations. It strengthens and improves the voice, and eliminates throat ailments.

Notes:

Brahmari pranayama induces a meditative state by harmonizing the mind and directing the awareness inwards. The vibrations of the sound create a soothing effect on the mind and the nervous system. The word Brahmari means "bee" and the practice is so-called because a sound is produced, which imitates that of the black bee.

Warning:

People suffering from severe ear infections should not practice this pranayama until the infection has been cured.

5) Bhastrika Pranayama:

How to do it:

- Sit in any comfortable meditation asana, preferably Padmasana, Vajrasana, Sukhasana, with hands resting on knees.
- Keep the head and the spine upright, close the eyes and relax.
- Inhale and exhale at the speed of approximately one breath per second.
- The number of respiration may be increased to 10 in the beginning to a maximum of 30 to 40 respirations.
- Inhalation and exhalation must be equal.
- Practice up to 5 rounds.

Bhastrika is a dynamic practice requiring large generation of physical energy. Beginners are advised to take a short rest after each round. Bhastrika may be practiced at three different breath levels: slow, medium and fast, depending on the capacity of the practitioner.

Benefits:

Bhastrika pranayama burns up the toxins. Because of the rapid exchange of the air in the lungs, there is an increase in the exchange of oxygen and carbon dioxide into and out of blood stream. This stimulates the metabolic rate, producing heat and flushing out wastes and toxins from the system and helps reducing the excess fat.

It balances and strengthens the nervous system, inducing peace and tranquility.

Bhastrika reduces the level of carbon dioxide in the lungs. It is an excellent practice for the asthmatics and for those suffering from other lung disorders.

Note:

The word Bhastrika means "bellows" in Sanskrit language. In this pranayama, the air is drawn forcefully in and out of the lungs, like by the bellows of a village blacksmith. The bellows increases the flow of the air into the fire, producing more heat. Similarly, Bhastrika pranayama increases the flow of air into the body to produce inner heat at both the physical and subtle levels, stoking the inner fire of mind/body.

Warning:

Bhastrika should not be practiced by people who suffer from high blood pressure, heart disease, hernia, gastric ulcer, stroke, epilepsy or vertigo.

6) Seetkari Pranayama (hissing breath):

How to do it:

- Sit in any comfortable meditation posture with hands on the knees.
- Close the eyes and relax the whole body.
- Hold the teeth lightly together. Separate the lips, exposing the teeth.

- The tongue may be kept flat or folded. Breath in slowly and deeply through the teeth.
- At the end of the inhalation, close the mouth and breath out slowly through the nose, in a slow motion.
- Practice 8 to 10 rounds.

Awareness:

Keep attention on the hissing sound while breathing in. Observe and feel the coolness inside the body.

Benefits:

The practice of this pranayama cools the body and the mind as well. It keeps teeth and gums healthy. It cools and reduces mental and emotional excitation, and encourages the free flow of prana throughout the body. It gives control over hunger and thirst, and generates a feeling of satisfaction. It helps reduce blood pressure and acid in the stomach.

8

Meditation

When the surface of the water of a lake is still, one can see the bottom of the lake very clearly. This is impossible when the surface is agitated by waves. In the same way, when the mind is still, with no thoughts or desires, one can see the "Self"; the process to achieve this is called "Yoga".

The mind is one sort of lifeless substance. It is not conscious. Therefore no thought protrudes in mind itself nor does the mind itself raise any thought. Conscious soul is the driver of this insentient mind. When conscious soul desires to raise any kind of virtuous or non-virtuous thought in mind, then and then only the thought related to that subject protrudes.

There are four types of thought which disturb our mind in our daily life, in one or the other way.

- Thoughts of harming someone,
- Thoughts of Jealousy,
- Thoughts of doubts and uncertainty,
- Thoughts of attachments.

If we analyze our thoughts which bother us during the day, most probably they will fit in the any of above four categories.

We can control the mental agitation by two means: by concentrating the mind either externally or internally. Internally, we focus on the "Self" or the consciousness of "I am". Externally, we focus on anything other than the "Self" or "I am".

When we take up some recreation on putting the ball into the hole (golf), the other thoughts are slowed down or stilled. We feel we have played a good game when we have achieved perfect concentration. The happiness we experience comes, not because the ball is being put in the hole eighteen times, but because we have achieved the perfect concentration eighteen times. At that time, all the worries and problems of the world disappear.

The mental ability to concentrate on self is inherent to all; it is not extraordinary or mysterious. Meditation is not something that a Yogi has to teach you; you already have the ability to shut out the thoughts.

The only difference between this and meditation (the positive way), is that, generally, we have learned to focus the mind externally on objects. When the mind is fully concentrated, time passes unnoticed, as if it did not exist. When the mind is focused, there is no time! Time is nothing but a modification of the mind.

All happiness achieved through the mind is temporary and brief; it is limited by nature. To achieve that state of lasting happiness and absolute peace, we must first know how to calm the mind, to concentrate and go beyond the mind. By turning the mind's concentration inward, upon the self, we can deepen that experience of perfect concentration. This is called the real state of Meditation.

The Inside of Meditation

Meditation is an experience that cannot be described, just as colors cannot be described to a blind man. All ordinary experiences are limited by Time, Space and Causation. Our normal awareness and understanding do not transcend these bounds.

Finite experience, which is measured in terms of past, present and future, cannot be transcendental. Concepts of time are illusory, for they have no permanence. The present, immeasurably small and fleeting, cannot be grasped. Past and future are non-existent in the present. We live in illusion.

The meditative state transcends all such limitations. In it, there is neither past nor future, but only the consciousness of "I am" in the eternal NOW. It is only possible when all mental modifications are stilled.

Each of our body cells is governed by the instinctive subconscious mind. They have both an individual and a collective consciousness. When the thoughts and desires pour into the body, the cells are activated; the body always obeys the group demand. It has been scientifically proved that positive thoughts bring positive result to cells. As meditation brings about a prolonged positive state of mind, it rejuvenates body cells and retards the decaying process and ageing.

How to Practice Meditation

Meditation is constant awareness of self. It has no technique and cannot be learnt from anyone else. No one else can teach you how to quiet the brain and control wandering thoughts. If you force the mind to be quiet and still, that is not meditation.

Meditation begins when you learn to listen to yourself, to enquire, observe and watch. There has to be constant awareness. Meditation is not an activity of isolation. It is watching awareness of whatever is happening to you inwardly and also from outside.

Meditation is not separate from daily life but an essential and constant part of it. For meditation, do not go off to a corner of the room for ten minutes, then come out of it and describe your experience of seeing lights in darkness, hearing bells ringing, and smelling flowers in the breeze. This is simply delusion and an escape from reality. Meditation is something that should be done all day, every day. It is a part of your life, not something separate or anything different.

Teachers, gurus, priests or rishis cannot teach meditation. No outside authority is needed. All that is needed is total attention to whatever you are saying, doing or thinking. This total attention is meditation.

Meditation is self-awareness—the awareness of every thought, feeling and movement of the conscious and unconscious mind. Mediation is the understanding of everything that lies beyond thought and feeling. And this is, perhaps, the most difficult of all the ways to meditate. To be conscious at all times of everything you are doing, thinking, feeling is the meditation.

Solitude is not required, nor is it necessary. What is required is one's consciousness for being ever centered in the present. "Present moment, only moment". There is no past, no future—only NOW.

Meditating should be in the secret recess of your heart and mind. If you follow a particular system or method, that would bind you down. Simply being aware of every thought and feeling releases you from time and thought.

In meditation, the mind is empty of both past and future and is therefore timeless.

Meditation begins with the mind, not with the body. Concentration and rigidly held posture makes it difficult to practice constant awareness that is beyond imagination or desire. Our minds are time-based. If we can simply watch our minds and bodies without judging or assessing or trying to understand, then the mind becomes naturally silent, without suppression or control.

To such a mind there is no time, and therefore living has quite a different meaning.

Some truth about Meditation

The most effective times are early dawn and dusk, when the atmosphere is charged with special spiritual force. If it is not feasible to sit for meditation at these times, choose an hour when you are not involved in daily activities, and a time when the mind is apt to be calm.

Consciously regulate the breath. Begin with five minutes of deep abdominal breathing to bring oxygen to the brain. Then slow it down to an imperceptible rate.

Keep the breathing rhythmic, inhale for three seconds and exhale for three seconds. Regulation of breath also regulates the flow of prana, the vital energy to body.

Allow the mind to wander at first. It will jump around, but will eventually become concentrated, along with the concentration of prana. Do not force the mind to be still, as this will set in motion additional brain waves, hindering meditation.

If you meditate for half an hour daily, you will be able to face life with peace and spiritual strength. Meditation is the most powerful mental and nerve tonic. Divine energy freely flows to the adept during meditation, and exerts a benign influence on the mind, nerves, sense organs and body. It opens the door to intuitive knowledge and realms of eternal bliss. The mind becomes calm and steady.

The mind is an instrument in the hands of the soul, and it is constantly vacillating from one subject to another. In our ordinary state when the mind is attached intently to one organ, say, that of hearing while listening to music, it may not perceive through the other organs like the eyes, though they may be open. But the perfected mind can be attached to all the organs simultaneously. It has the reflexive power of looking back into its own depth. By concentrating all the powers of mind and turning them inward, we seek to know what is happening inside.

A simple way of meditation

To be independent of influences is called Pratyahara or abstinence. Pratyahara is a natural process and it has nothing to do with exertion or strain. You do not try to force disturbances to leave your mind. On the contrary, you allow your mind to be occupied with them until the mind is satisfied—while all along you remain the silent witness.

When you try to stop thoughts and disturbances from going through your mind, they will only return to bother you. Pratyahara is a method which complies with the mind's habitual way of reacting. Therefore, as a necessary basis for relaxing the mind, you learn to use the methods of Pratyahara; when the needs of your mind are satisfied, you will be able to concentrate with greater ease.

Following are the four phases of action to practice meditation:

Phase 1:

- Sit in sukhasana and close the eyes.
- Relax the whole body.

- Listen to all the surrounding sounds. Listen to all of them—without discriminating—as a whole, all at the same time.
- Observe the thoughts enter and leaving your mind.
- Do not try to force disturbances to leave your mind.
- Easy they come, easy they will go.
- You can "warm up" with a couple of deep and smooth breaths like Ujjayi pranayama or Nadi Shodhana.

Phase 2:

- Breath through your nose. Focus on your breath—"cool air in, warm air out". If the mind wanders, gently bring it back to the breath. Count your breaths for easy concentration.
- Observe and analyze the thoughts entering the mind.
- Find out about the type of thoughts, like attachment, harming someone, jealousy, doubts and uncertainty.
- Think about how much they bother you, and about what you get after thinking like that.

Phase 3:

- After a few days of practice, start asking questions to yourself. Your mind will ask the question and your soul will answer it. After some time of practice, there will be no question and no answer, only silence.
- This question and answer session will take you to the deep awareness of your existence.
- Slowly and steadily, those harmful thoughts will start disappearing from your mind. Only thoughts of happiness and joy will wander through your mind.
- Mind will come to total calmness.

Mediation is just like that—easy and enjoyable. No force and no discrimination. Just observe and enjoy.

Start with a 5-10 minute meditation, and work your way up to 15, 20, 30 minutes or more. You can practice the meditation at any where and at any time when ever you have time.

9

Relaxation: To Recharge the Mind and the Body

When the body and the mind are constantly overworked, their natural efficiency to perform work diminishes. Modern social life, food eating habits, work culture and even the so-called entertainment, such as disco dancing, make it difficult for modern people to relax and relieve.

Many even forget that rest and relaxation are nature's way of recharging the mind and the soul. Even while trying to rest, the average person expends a lot of physical and mental energy through tension. Much of the body's energy is wasted unnecessarily.

Real relaxation actually strengthens our immune system and protects us from many diseases like hypertension, heart attacks and ulcers. Relaxation increases efficiency, enhances energy and vitality.

Most people think that they are relaxing when they watch TV or drink a glass of wine. Indeed, there is some alleviation of stress in both these activities but the basic tension returns as soon as the TV is switched off or the glass of wine is drained.

Real relaxation is much more than this. The muscles are soft and without tension and brain waves slow down to a serene state of emotional and mental calm. This is the Alpha state in which the brain's rhythm slows down to 8 to 14 cycles per second; two halves of the brain is in balance and we are less aware of the body or our surroundings. In this state the immune system is strengthened, the body is better able to heal itself and the mind is able to be both creative and intuitive.

To get into the state of deep relaxation, one needs to utilize the three S's: Silence, Stillness and Solitude—and avail of Shavasana or what is called dead body posture.

More of our energy is spent in keeping the muscles in continual readiness for work than it is spent in the actual useful work done. In order to regulate and balance the work of the body and mind, it is best to learn to economize the energy produced by our body. This may be done by learning to relax.

It may be remembered that in the course of one day, our body usually produces all the substances and energy necessary for the next day. But it often happens that all these substances and energy may be consumed, within a few minutes, by bad moods, anger, injury or intense irritation. The process of eruption and repression of violent emotions often grows into a regular habit. The result is disastrous, not only for the body but also for the mind.

During complete relaxation, there is practically no energy or "Prana" being consumed, although a little of it is keeping the body in normal condition while its remaining portion is being stored and conserved.

In order to achieve perfect relaxation, three methods are used by yogis: "Physical", "Mental", and "Spiritual".

Physical Relaxation

We know that every action is the result of thought. Just as the mind sends a message to the muscles ordering them to contract, the mind may also send another message to bring the relaxation to the tired muscles.

The correct practice of Shavasana or the Dead Man's Posture is good for both body and mind. Learning to die while you live is good for body and mind. It also opens the gates to spiritual well-being..

Physical relaxation first begins with the toes and then moves upward. The autosuggestion passes through the muscles and reaches the eyes and ears at the top. Then, slowly, messages are sent to the kidneys, liver and the other internal organs.

Ten minutes of the relaxation through Shavasana after asanas, or pranayama or meditation gives unbelievable benefits to body and mind. Even when you feel tired or come under pressure due to job related dead line or any other mental irritation, practice Shavasana to relax and relieve.

Mental Relaxation

When experiencing mental tension, it is advisable to breath slowly and rhythmically for a few minutes. Soon the mind will become calm. You may experience a kind of floating sensation.

Spiritual Relaxation

However one may try to relax the mind, all tensions and worries cannot be completely removed until one reaches spiritual relaxation.

As long as a person identifies with the body and the mind, there will be worries, sorrows, anxieties, fear and anger. These emotions, in turn, bring tension. Yogis know that unless a person withdraws from the body/mind idea and separate himself from the ego-consciousness, there is no way of obtaining complete relaxation.

The yogi identifies himself with the all-pervading, all-powerful, all-peaceful and joyful self, or pure consciousness within. He knows that the source of all power, knowledge, peace and strength is in the self, not in the body. We tune to this by asserting the real nature, that is, "I am that pure consciousness or self". This identification with the self completes the process of relaxation.

Systematically we relax first the respiratory system, then the muscles, the joints, the blood circulation, the brain, and the eyes—the entire physical body.

This psychosomatic relaxation is not just an ordinary relaxation technique. It aims at achieving physical, mental and emotional equilibrium.

It is a doorway to the meditative state. When harmony pervades between the inner and the outer reality, your mind becomes more flexible—after all what is the use of making a resolution if your subconscious mind resists?

Yog Nidra

Yog Nidra (Deep Relaxation) is the method that allows you a maximum relaxation in a minimum of time. One hour of Yoga Nidra is equivalent to four hours of sleep and is often an effective cure for insomnia. You can use Yoga Nidra with the help of a guided recording on a CD or a tape. The instructions given by this CD or tape are to be followed while lying down in Shavasana.

Yoga Nidra is not only for those who are worn out or mentally tense but also for those who are tired of inactivity. With Yoga Nidra, you begin to develop a state of inner awareness and deep calm. The Yoga Nidra can be practiced after doing asanas, pranayama, meditation or aerobic exercise. Yoga Nidra is good after intensive physical or mental work. This is helpful in case of depression, worries or tension.

If a prerecorded CD or tape is not available, then you can practice by yourself. Here are step by step instructions for how to fall into Yog Nidra.

1. Make sure the room is quiet and slightly dark.

2. Lie down on a bed sheet on the floor, comfortably.

3. Take the shavasana position. Close eyes and relax the whole body.

4. Observe the breathing. Breathing should be slow and minimal.

5. No movement, and observe the complete silence, both outside and inside.

6. Bring your attention towards the toes. Give some movement to the toes. Then relax the toes and the feet. Imagine how the toes and the feet look and how useful they are to you in walking. Remember their importance in your life.

7. After that, turn your attention to the knees, and follow the same process as above, going from one organ to one after another upto the head and paying attention to every joints, organs, ears, nose, lips, eyes, and anything that serves you to live life.

8. The whole process should be slow and steady, with 100% involvement.

9. At the end, stay for a few minutes in relax position and then open the eyes slowly.

It may be little difficult to sleep and practice like that but it will be normal after the practice of a few sessions. If a tape or a cd for Yog Nidra is available from any reliable source, try to use it.

10

Ayurveda: A complete way of living

More than 5,000 years ago, the great seers of ancient India studied the fundamentals of life and organized them into a healing system called Ayurveda. This system—which in Sanskrit means "science of life"—is essentially an operating manual for the body, the mind, and the spirit.

The original indigenous therapy, Ayurveda, is a combination of two words "Ayur" denoting life and "Veda" denoting knowledge. Practiced since ancient times, Ayurveda has been a natural system of medicine. Ayurveda is not merely a therapy but a complete way of living.

Ayurveda can treat ailments like obesity, diabetes, hypertension, heart disease, anorexia, arthritis, asthma addictions, Alzheimer's disease, gastrointestinal disorder, bronchitis, impotence, multiple sclerosis and osteoporosis, among others. Ill-health is a result of imbalance of elements and soul, which is corrected by natural drugs like herbs, minerals, metals, and food.

Ayurveda, the classic system of Indian medicine, classifies people, as well as food into three categories according to their nature. According to the Ayurvedic system, people are born with a particular constitution (or prakruti) that defines their baseline of health.

Three Vital Energies or Doshas:

An individual's constitution is made up of a delicate balance of three vital energies, or doshas, known as **vata** (air, dry and light), **pitta** (fire, hot and oily), and **kapha** (water, cold and moist). In Ayurveda, the individual's diet should be tailored to the individual's constitution to keep these doshas in balance. These doshas govern all the psychological, physiological, and patho-physiological functions of mind and body; and they are the basis for diagnosing illness.

The three doshas are actually three processes inside the body system. Vata is the process of movement, and its catabolic energy breaks down the matter. Pitta is a process of metabolism that creates heat and energy in much the same way that fire breaks down a log. Kapha is dense, heavy matter that stores energy, like the fat and padding in our bodies.

Balancing of these three doshas is the actual health of man. Any imbalance between these three doshas can create disturbances inside the body, resulting in ill health.

Food as Medicine:

Some foods which are recommended for a particular ayurvedic constitution may not be suitable for another; for example, while milk, a sattvic food, is generally good for Pitta constitution; it may not suit someone with a Kapha constitution. The ideal ayurvedic diet also changes, depending on the time of the year.

Foods are also classified as vata, pitta, and kapha, and they either decrease or aggravate a person's doshas. The aggravation of the doshas goes along with ill health, as either cause or result. Food should have a neutralizing effect on the doshas and not that of aggravating them.

Eating foods that complement your constitution helps to maintain the body's balance. An illness, whether a common cold or a serious disease, indicates that the doshas are out of balance, a condition that is worsened by eating foods that clash with your dosha.

According to Ayurveda, you are ingesting more than just food when you eat. As you eat, you take into yourself the subtle influences attached to the food and prana as well as the physical form of the food. Even the stages of production to which food is subjected affect its qualities. Food is a part of the dynamic dance of life; and its qualities, both obvious and subtle, affect your well-being.

The basic Ayurvedic diet consists of whole, fresh foods in season, with vegetables forming between 20 and 40 percent of the diet. Usually, only a quarter of the foods are eaten raw; the rest are cooked. An ideal Ayurvedic diet is different for each person, based on the individual's own blend of vata, pitta, and kapha. The process of constructing a personalized diet is best done by observing one's body requirement and changes.

Ayurveda is not intellectual. It is a practice that uses your intuition, the creative aspect of your mind, your own body knowledge. The bottom line in Ayurveda is relying on what your body tells you and not on what a theory, or a book, or a practitioner tells you. Ayurveda is just a framework for understanding your own body nature.

When a person has cold and has congestion in the chest, that congestion is due to kapha (Cough). In order to reduce the kapha, pitta needs to be increased. Pitta is heat, so eating hot foods, like ginger, will reduce the congestion. Continuing to eat kapha foods like ice cream, or drinking cold water, will increase the congestion.

Ayurveda diet is a constant source of inspiration. The following Ayurvedic recipes are best against the symptoms of cold and flu.

Tea for Colds

- 1 tablespoonful of grated fresh ginger root
- 1 tablespoonful of dried hibiscus flowers (from a health food or a herb store)
- 1 to 2 sticks of cinnamon
- Put ginger, hibiscus flowers, and cinnamon sticks in 3 cups of boiling water.
- Simmer for several minutes, and then turn off the heat, and cover for five minutes. Sweeten with fresh orange juice or honey.

Sore Throat Gargle

This very traditional remedy is less palatable and more antiseptic than the tea, but it strengthens the throat tissue.

- 1 teaspoonful of turmeric powder
- Dissolve the turmeric powder in hot water. Gargle with it, and then swallow.

Kichari

Kichari (Indian Gujarati food) is the best food for those recovering from illness, as it is very healing and easy to digest.

1 tablespoonful of ghee, 6 ounces of basmati rice, 3 teaspoonfuls of cumin seeds, 3 teaspoonfuls of coriander seeds, 3 teaspoonfuls of fennel seeds, 1/2 teaspoonful of turmeric powder, 3 ounces of split yellow mung beans (dal), vegetables appropriate to your doshas

- Wash rice and beans together under cold water.

- Melt ghee in a pan, and then add fennel seeds. Cook for one minute. Add cumin, coriander, and turmeric, and the rice and beans.

- Stir so that the mixture is coated with ghee. Add hot water upto a two-inch level. Then cover the mixture. Bring it to a boil; lower the heat and allow to simmer, stirring the mixture occasionally.

- Add a little more water if you do not want the pan to dry out while the food is being cooked.

- Add diced vegetables, starting with root vegetables. Leafy vegetables like spinach, should be added toward the end of the cooking time.

- The dish is cooked when most of the water has evaporated and the grains are soft and slightly mushy.

This food is most suitable even during illness and after illness.

Herbals and Spices:

For many years, Ayurveda has described numerous herbals and spices and their benefits in maintaining health. Herbals and spices, when taken as part of food, boost up immune system, increase vitality power, and give protection against a deadly disease like Cancer, Alzheimer, Hyper tension. These herbals are useful in curing some day-to-day diseases and they work very well in place of medicines.

The list of herbals and spices is very long. A few of them are Turmeric, Garlic, Ginger, Dry Ginger, Chillies, Coriander seeds and leaves, Basil leaves, Caraway, Black pepper, Asafetida, Clove, Niger or Seasamum, Cinnamon, Nutmeg, Cumin seeds, Saffron, Camphor, Phyllenthus emblica, Buck wheat, Mustard, Castor seed, Honey, Sulphur, Menthol, etc. We hardly use these useful herbals and spices in our daily food. These wonderful products of nature are made to protect our body from different viruses and bacteria.

Few herbals with their medical values are described here. Readers who are interested should read more about these products from other sources.

Turmeric: Turmeric is one of the best blood purifiers. It also cures cough, and smoothens the throat. It also removes skin disease, and beautifies the skin. Fresh turmeric should be used as part of salad, with lemon and slight salt on it.

Garlic: It is most helpful in reducing cholesterol in blood, and protects us from heart attack. It helps in maintaining body temperature, and is recommended against TB bacteria or bacilli.

Ginger: It promotes appetite and is helpful in winter time. It boosts up our immune system and cleans up our body.

Oil massage for body:

Many of the treatments in Ayurveda are intended to create deep peace and relaxation. In one, oil massage with warm sesame oil to body for 15 minutes, creates a state similar to that achieved in mediation.

Due to oil massage, veins, which carry blood inside the body, become flexible, and accumulated fat deposits inside the veins get cleared. Body organs, joints, skin, bones, tissues and millions of cells get massage to work efficiently.

Seasamum or Mustard oil is the best for massage. Also Mahanarayan oil, produced by many ayurvedic medicine manufacturers in India, is good for body massage. Use anyone of them for self-massaging for about 5 to 10 minutes every morning before bath or shower.

11

Daily Routine: A day with Yogic Life

A normal day should begin between 5:00 a.m. and 5:30a.m. Getting up early morning before sunrise is best for health. Morning time is really quiet and very serene for practicing yogas and other exercises.

As we all know that we have limited numbers of days to spend in life, so each and every day and every moment is important to us. Typical day of the yogic day of life looks something like this. It may have some changes according to the situation and surroundings of our life. Let us assume that a typical day starts at 5:30a.m.

Daily Routine

- Wake up at 5:30a.m. This can be adjusted as per one's requirement.

- Drink 2 to 4 glasses of luke-warm water immediately after getting up from the bed.

- Finish the cleaning activities like brushing teeth, bowels motion, etc. but do not take a bath. The time is 5:45a.m.

- Do some of the asanas (Yogic exercise) for 30 minutes as discussed.

- Take special juice extracted from Ginger, Turmeric, Phyllenthus emblica (Amala, available in an Indian Grocery store as fresh fruit; if this is not available, then use a few drops of fresh lemon) with one teaspoonful of honey. Details about this are given in Chapter No. 3.

- Take your bath. The time is 6:45 a.m.
- Get ready for Pranayama followed by Meditation. The time is 7:15 a.m.
- Have breakfast and get ready for work at 7:30a.m.
- Take a glass of water or fresh fruit juice at 9:00a.m.
- Drink again a glass of water between 10:00 a.m. and 11:00 a.m.
- Take lunch between 12 noon and 1:00 p.m.
- Drink a glass of water at 2:30p.m.
- Have afternoon snacks between 3:30 to 4:00 p.m. Prefer fresh fruits or juice to tea or coffee.
- Drink a glass of water each at 5:00 p.m. and 6:00 p.m. Observe the 1 hour gap before and after any food intake.
- Take evening dinner between 7:00 p.m. and 8:00 p.m.
- Before going to bed, take trifala powder or a trifala tablet with water. Both are made of herbals and are innocent to stomach.
- Clean the teeth before going to bed. Use Ayurvedic powder to clean the teeth. Modern toothpastes contain many chemicals, and they can upset the digestive system. At least use tooth powder in the night time.
- Do not take food after 10:00 p.m. under any circumstances. Food eaten after 10 p.m. generates toxins in body rather than provide any useful nutrition.
- Wash the eyes with cold water 4 to 6 times a day. This practice will delay the eye disease like glaucoma or cataract.
- Go to bed at 10:00 p.m. Sound sleep is another requirement for long and happy life. Look at the birds and animals, they follow

night sleep schedule very punctually. Night time is designed by God for sleep. During sleep many repairing and recharging activities are going on inside the body.

The above routine is ideal to get longevity and happiness. An individual can make certain changes according to his or her own time schedule if any time is not suitable to follow this routine strictly. It is all right if certain compromise and flexibility are made in this routine.

But under normal conditions, the above routine should be followed to get the desired results. It is also important that sooner you start in the early life, better it will be. To live for 100 years happily and healthily is not impossible provided you implement everything described in this book, faithfully.

Human body has a wonderful and unique immune system, which corrects minor mistakes made by us off and on.

Yogic sleep

Sleep is the most important part of daily routine, in order to be healthy and happy. We spend almost one third of our life span in just sleeping. Sleep has as much importance as food. During sleep, our body makes necessary repair and restoration work inside.

Insomnia is the most well-know problem in this hectic world. Sleep disorder hurt us personally and professionally.

Never sleep with head covered by a bed sheet or blanket. Our body is a kind of factory, and it is continuously emitting carbon dioxide while it is breathing out. If we cover our face with a bed sheet, we inhale stale carbon dioxide again into our body. Body can not do the required restoration work of cells, tissues and other important body organs due to lack of fresh oxygen. After enough sleep, we can not feel fresh and energetic due to this wrong practice of sleeping.

We sometimes experience in our life uneasiness, lack of concentration, tireness due to shortage of sleep. Ayurveda asserts that sleep is essential for longevity. To live long and happy, we must have natural sound sleep without any external, artificial help. Please stay away from any sleeping pills or tranquilizers to get sleep. They harm our body more than they benefit.

Here are a few yogic remedies to obtain natural and sound sleep.

1. The first and foremost requirement for sound sleep is punctuality in timing. Try to go to bed at the same time every night and get up at the same time every morning.

2. Bedroom should be dark enough. If outside temperature permits, keep windows open to let the fresh air in.

3. Do not eat heavy and plenty of food for dinner. Light food is the best bet for sound sleep. Excess generation of gas inside the body is the prime reason for sleepless nights.

4. There should be the gap of at least 2 to 3 hours between dinner and going to bed.

5. Take shower of warm water just before sleep time.

6. Make a note of work that you want to do the next morning, so that the mind will be free from the stress of remembering the next-day work.

7. Practice the Ujjayi pranayama for about 5 minutes before going to bed.

8. Count 100 in mind and then count in the reverse order. This will help you fall sleep unnoticed.

9. Even after that if you are not able to sleep, then close the eyes and sit straight if a particular thought bothers you in getting sleep. Start meditation and think politely about that thought.

10. Health and Fear are the two main reasons for sleepless nights. You will be in glowing health if you sincerely practice whatever is mentioned in this book. As you learn the art of mediation, fear will disappear from mind at the time of sleep. Fear of finance, fear of job related work, fear of social commitments are the few types of fear troubling your mind at the time of going to bed. This state of mind does not allow you to fall asleep soon. With the help of Yoga and pranayama, you will be able to control any kind of fear.

12

Be Happy—Be Healthy: Do not worry

"Enjoy the life, because there is plenty of time to be dead"

What is the ultimate desire of mankind? The simple answer is "to be happy". We all want to be happy. At least, we all say "yes, we do want to be happy". We all know and we all are trying all our life to achieve that. Then another question is how to be happy. Can we be happy by owning a big house, a luxurious car, a fat bank balance or any other material facilities?

The straight answer is "no". To get happiness, first we must have peace of mind, and the peaceful mind will reside only in a healthy body.

This is the only life we have got. It is up to us how to live, to get maximum happiness or to waste it just for nothing. Just think of how many human beings have visited this planet so far. We can count the population on this planet, but we have no idea as to how many have come to this planet and have gone out of this world for eternal.

Let us take a common example of modern life. Say, one of our friends bought some stock shares. After some time, he finds that the share prices have gone up. The prices of this particular stock had been going up and our friend was getting happy because his investment value was increasing day after day. Actually he did not sell any stock so he did not receive any money. While he is thinking that his share holding is increasing in value, happy waves are generated in his mind. Theses happy waves are the real happiness. The state of mind ensures real happiness and unhappiness. Remember: we are what we think.

After a few days, that same stock is going in the reverse direction. In a few days, it loses whatever it had gained in the last few days. Our friend starts blaming himself. He thinks he should have sold the stock at that moment. Due to this thinking, unhappy waves are generated in his mind. This is the state of unhappiness where there is no loss of money. The psyche ensures either of the states of our mind.

In both instances, our friend actually did not gain or lose anything. Everything was just on paper and still he became happy at one moment and unhappy at the other moment. Our whole life goes the roller coaster way or like a pendulum. From time to time our mind generates waves of pains and gains, joy and jealousy, happiness and harming, security and sorrow. It is simply the state of mind. Let the mind remain calm and quiet so that no other outside events can disturb our mind. To learn how to get mind calmed in any situation, we should learn Yoga and practice it regularly.

Each of us has been given the gift of life fuelled by the life-force or prana. Have we ever wondered why we sometimes feel low, drained, and energyless? We might feel so after a stressful period—because of trying circumstances, a spell of hectic work or sudden trauma. Often, we are unable to pinpoint a reason for it. And for some of us it may become a state of being; a joyless, purposeless existence. "A healthy body with a peaceful mind leads to a happy life." Let us understand this combination and take a look at following thoughts, and be happy.

Worship, not worry:

> Ah, fill the cup; what boots it to repeat
> How time is slipping underneath our feet,
> Unborn tomorrow and dead yesterday to beat,
> Why fret about them if Today is so sweet?

Do not worry, Be happy—Be healthy. A funeral pyre burns the dead people, but worries burn the living people. Worries never allow you to live in the present moments. It always takes you to either in the past or in the future. Worry causes fear, anxiety, tension and stress. These emotions deplete energy and weaken the immune system.

If worry drains you with fears of the future, then hurt, resentment and regret keep you chained to the past. As you nourish the memories of the people who have hurt you or let you down, of circumstances that have betrayed your expectations, or of unfulfilled dreams, you are only draining energy to something that is, in fact, dead and gone. You can still remember and talk about it with tears in your eyes. The person, meanwhile, is no longer a part of your life; he may even have passed on or out but you continue to leak energy to this thought.

It would be sensible to look at life as a long chain of surprises. So live it sportingly. The goal of life is not to achieve some mythical point of perfect materialism. The goal of life is simply to work hard at becoming better today than you were yesterday. In life there are no wars to be won, only battles to be fought—personal, physical, social, psychological and spiritual.

In our efforts to live life sensibly, God plays the role of the eternal comrade, the invisible companion, the universal friend. Prayer and worship give serenity in our life, calm down the mind and bring complete silence in thoughts. Prayer, in any form of classic music with devotional song for God, is a real approach to God. By listening to the prayer, the mind comes to a silence state and worries disappear just like vapor.

Health or Wealth:

There is always a mental confusion about whether or not health is better than wealth. Wealth is required to live a decent life but without health, there is no joy or happiness in life. You can buy a costly bedroom, but not sound sleep; can buy delicious food, but not appetite. If you are healthy, chances are that you might earn money but if you are wealthy, it is not necessary that you will be healthy unless you maintain your health. So health is primary and wealth is secondary if you want to be a discriminatory person in this respect.

Most people see money as the starting point for exchange, a means to acquiring goods and services. To be able to acquire more and more of goods and services, they strive to accumulate more and more money, working extra hours. They usually forget that money comes at a real price. Money is not the only and the first point of exchange. When they are struggling to earn money, they are exchanging their good life for money.

Pursuit of money can become an end in itself. It can distort all values, and make you blind to the basic purpose of life. Most of our life is spent in the pursuit of money. We often compare our material possessions in terms of money. Actually it should be equivalent to the number of years we spend to earn money. We must understand how to minimize the portion of the time devoted to organizing food, clothing and shelter, so that the bulk of the prime time is available for attending to a higher value in life.

The bottom line is that we should not destroy our health while earning wealth. Remember that our wealth is not our health but our health is our wealth.

Seven bad-habits of most of the unhappy people:

1. Hatred: You should not hate any people from any community, color, caste, creed or origin of a country. Love all and be a real cosmopolitan. No matter who they are, they are all human beings and visit this planet for a short time. Hatredness works like termites. It destroys our body slowly and steadily as termites destroy the wood on long run.

2. Anger: Anger is a violent emotion. It takes just a fraction of a moment to rise, surge and take complete possession of a person and shake his physical, mental and emotional balance. Angry persons often use insulting, abusive and humiliating language to their colleagues, friends and relatives, resulting in the bitter relations and also in the breakdown of a family. It destroys the happiness of life and invites many kinds of diseases.

3. Dishonesty: Honesty is the best policy and principle. It gives inner satisfaction and self-fulfilment. Now if you behave dishonest in your daily life with your family, friends, colleague or your clients, your warm relations will destroy with them. You will feel lonely and withdrawn from all people surroundings your life.

4. Selfishness: This brings negative thoughts inside the mind and disturbs inner peace.

5. Jealousy: This bad habit forces you to live the life beyond your reach and it traps you in debt. Be happy in what you have, and avoid comparison with peers.

6. Laziness: Do your job and duty sincerely. Laziness in doing an exercise, house work, and job related work brings misery and disputes.

7. Greed: This always keeps you in a state of anxiety and worries because, no matter how much you earn, you are not going to satisfy yourself. Sky is the only limit for greedy people. You should draw the line of "enough is enough."

Seven good-habits of most of the happy people:

1. Satisfaction: The more you are satisfied, the closer will come peace and happiness to you. This is the most important virtue to be happy in this material world.

2. Mercy: Mercy on the hungry, the poor, the insane, the helpless and the disabled people.

3. Control on food: Food is a fuel to body and not the fun in eating. Always keep in mind that it is food which is responsible for diseases of modern day life style.

4. Enough physical work: As long as you eat food, you must work physically and mentally.

5. Trust in God: Right or wrong, good or bad, you must have faith in Him. So accept the events as they happen.

6. Simple life and high thinking: It protects you from depression and unwarranted situation.

7. Live and let live: We are all creatures of the same God. Everyone has a right to survive and live his/her own life. Weaker or stronger, poor or rich, here or there, we all belong to the same planet.

Success and Spirituality

We all are looking for success. What do we think is success? The parameters of success are changing with times. A few years ago, may be, a couple of decades ago-wearing a lot of jewellery was considered a parameter of success. Different countries and different people had their own parameters of success at that time. Today, that is not so. Today, the sign of lasting smile, confidence in life, and a sense of belonging to everybody around are the real success and aim of life.

Life is made of matter and spirit. Matter is—amino acids, proteins, bones, blood, flesh, etc. Spirit is made up of enthusiasm, joy, love, beauty in life. We need food for stomach, taste for tongue, beauty for eyes, and fun for celebration. All these are a part of our life. Spirituality is something that encompasses all these avenues—value system, human value, compassion, caring, sharing—all are components of spirituality. Spirituality is not just sitting and doing some practice. Spirituality is a value system; it is a way of life; it is a specific state of a healthy mind.

Quality of our life is determined by the state of our mind. Health is much more than absence of illness. Success is something beyond money in the bank or material possessions. The status we have attained and the comforts of home and family are no guarantee of happiness. The true value of our own inner joy of life lies in how much we share it with others. Let us ask these questions to ourselves and try to get their answers, too. At the end, we will be able to find out that real success lies in the positive values in human life. Be introspective and try to find out answers to these questions:

- Are you squeezing yourself with stress and tension most of the time?
- Can you spend enough time for yourself and for your family?
- How long are you going to live?
- What do you want to accomplish in the remaining years of your life?

Forget and Forgive:

Life is the sequence of happy and unhappy events and moments. Many times during course of the time in life, certain events and moments happen against our wishes. We may not like them but they become part of our life for rest of our life. Their memories give us pain and suffering, anger and agitation, sorry and sorrow.

We should learn to forget and forgive. If someone, whom you trust very much, has betray you or your dearest and nearest insult you, best way to be happy is forget about what happen to you and forgive him who behaved like that with you.

Forget and forgive are two magic words worth implementing in our life. They are capable of bringing back our lost happiness and disappeared smiles on our face.

Ego: Root of unhappiness

As described before, ego is a thin layer between us and soul (self). This thin and invisible layer is very difficult to break in but it is possible. Whoever is able to break this layer of ego, enjoy eternal happiness under any circumstances.

Different people have ego for different reasons like beauty, power, money, social status, education, knowledge, talent or skill, etc.

Look at the big and vast sandy desert. Pick up one small particle of sand, our earth is smaller than that small particle of sand in this universe. Is it possible to identify the location of our country, our town or our own house? The whole universe is so vast that our existence has no place in it. Still we live all our life in fake imagination that "I" am the superior than my surrounding people. All our life we live in false pride and unrealistic pretending.

Millions and billions of people had come and gone from this earth. There is no record for them. Still they all believed that they were number one in their field.

Because we are narrow-minded, we cannot be linked to the Almighty God. Only when egotism has been uprooted, do all the powers come from God and begin to flow unto us. If we want to be really happy, our ego should be at zero level. Always think that whoever we are and whatever we have, is gift of God. We are here to fulfill our duty and live happy and healthy life.

Positive Thinking and Attitude:

A glass is half full or half empty. If we think it is half full, then it is called positive thinking. It is all about seeing and thinking. When we see something and if we think positive about it, then it is positive thinking.

We always think and talk about others, but we never talk or think about ourselves. If we want to be happy and healthy, we must start talking to ourselves. That means trying to look inward and communicating with ourselves.

In the early morning, or, whenever you are alone at home, sit in the sukhasana pose. Close the eyes and start concentrating on your body. Slowly start asking the questions to yourself. Recollect any unpleasant or pleasant events you have experienced in your life time. What kind of the role did you play at that time? Did you hurt anybody by your words? How did you help someone and how did he appreciate your kind gesture? Who are you and why are you here? What do you want to do in the life and how long will you be here on this earth?

The more questions you ask yourself, the more deeply you will be able to understand yourself. After a few days of this practice, you will start realizing the weakness inside your mind and body. The first change will come in your behavior with your family and friends.

That will be the humble beginning of positive thinking and attitude. Positive thinking is required in order to be successful in life. Success brings happiness and happiness brings healthy life.

It is not what you do that counts but it is the attitude while doing a job that determines if the job is a karma yoga job, i.e. a liberating job, or, a binding job. Work is worship. Give your hands to work, and keep your mind fixed at the lotus feet of the Lord. Blessings are given not to the individual but to the efforts of the individual. Only if you start working, the blessing will begin to take effect. God will build a castle for you—not up in the air but within your heart, and it is you who have to lay a strong foundation for it.

Be the Best and Do Your Best

Whatever you have to do, just do it the best way. If you know a better way to serve, you must use it. Do not hold back because of the fear of effort or because of the fear of criticism. Do not work in a sloppy manner just because no one is watching you or because you feel the work is not for you. Give your best. Try to do such actions as can bring maximum good and minimum evil.

Right motive is same as right attitude. What matters is your real motive behind your actions and words. Your motive must be pure. Man generally plans to get the fruits of his work before he starts any kind of work. The mind is so framed that it cannot think of any kind of work without remuneration or reward. A selfish man cannot do any service. He will weigh the work and the money in a balance. Selfless service is unknown to him.

Often "duty" is referred to as "righteousness". You will incur demerit if you shun your duty. Your duty is towards God, or Self, or the Inner Teacher who teaches you through all the specific circumstances of your life as they appear.

Each job is a teacher of some sort. You can learn different skills by doing different jobs. Each job has different requirements in terms of time, degree of concentration, skills or experience, emotional input, physical energy, will. Try to do whatever job you are doing with full involvement.

Give up results and enjoy your work

God is the doer. You are not the doer. You are only an instrument. You do not know God's intentions or God's plans. God is the actor. The Self never acts but changes. The way to realize this truth is to constantly work for work's sake and let go the results, good or bad. It is the desire for action that binds the individual. It is the detachment from action that will dissolve the karmic seeds. Detachment from results also means detachment from the type of job itself. There is no job that is inferior or superior to another job. Do not be attached to your job. Be ready to give up your job if necessary.

Be 100% involved in whatever job you are doing, small or big. If you think about the results and outcomes of any task, you may not be able to perform your duty very well. Your attention will be on the results and eventually you will fail due to lack of concentration, and dedication and commitment.

Physical fitness, Emotional fitness:

To live a happy and healthy life, you should be physically fit as well as emotionally fit. Physical fitness is easily achievable, but emotional fitness is very difficult to achieve.

Emotions exercise great power and influence over our thoughts and actions. Negative emotions cause agitation, unrest, conflict, struggle, and frustration, resulting in unhappiness. Positive emotions, on the other hand, evoke feelings of calm, peace, happiness, and harmony. Let no thoughts can disturb you without your permission. You will be the complete in-charge of your mental state. Under any situation, waves of thoughts inside your mind should be uniform like a horizontal line on the screen of a cardiogram machine. No ups and down.

Whether some-one insults you, or, your best friend betrays you, the whole world is trying to prove that you are wrong even though you are right. If any situation agitates your mind, you should be calm and quiet. Nothing can bother you except yourself. This state makes you called emotionally fit. An agitated mind disturbs the biological balance of the inner body. If this kind of situation happens often, then the immune system becomes weak.

Laughing is the best medicine

Yes, when we laugh openly, our whole body shakes up and altogether about 70 different body organs participate in that action, provided that the laughing is purely innocent and not pointed towards anyone's origin, caste, color, religion, language, financial status, physical disability, etc.

Human being is the only creature which can laugh openly and totally. When we start laughing, the brain and the nervous system get extra oxygen in a short time. Brain tissues and cells release toxins from them.

Mind becomes relieved from stress and strain and face becomes more charming and cheerful. Lungs get stronger, deep breathing gets improved, heart beats become rapid, neck and shoulder get enough movements, and pancreas comes in shape. Laughing, as a matter of fact, is the best exercise.

Laughter comes out of health. It is an overflowing energy. That is why children can laugh and their laughter is total. Their whole body is involved when they laugh. In a spontaneous laughter, the noise of mind stops for a few precious moments, allowing us to experience mindlessness or meditation.

Laughing can add a few more friends, and people can trust you. It teaches you to work in group and share some private moments of your life.

If laughter is lost, everything is lost. Suddenly you lose the festivity of your being; you become colorless, in a way, dead. Laughing is the best medicine because it cures many unknown and undiagnosed diseases, at no cost. Be careful for time, location and situation for laughing. Laughter is good in a movie hall, but not in a church or a temple. If you use this medicine as much as you can, you will live long and happy.

Those who can laugh on themselves, live longer very easily.

Be responsible—Take responsibility

Responsibility is the power that makes you free from complaints. If you take responsibility for a certain task, immediately you stop complaining about it because now it is your responsibility to finish that task. Those who avoid any responsibility in their whole life and complain throughout their life become victims of negative thoughts and attitude.

Responsibility brings in our life some good virtues like dedication, accountability, punctuality, team spirit, integrity, self-esteem, consideration, fellowship. These good virtues build solid foundation of our well-being, ultimately leading to a happy and full life.

Prevention is better than cure:

An individual should maintain his health not by a bottle of medicine or through powders and pills or capsules but by a way of life which alone can promote health and prolong life or add life to his years and years to his life. Positive health is based on the salient principle of prevention. Prevention is better, easier, cheaper and safer than cure. Where as, curing is expensive, time-consuming and painful. The preventive outlook helps us in stopping the trouble before it starts or at the start. In health-matters, no reliance should be placed in the adage—"Never too late to mend". Intimate friendship with SEVEN doctors maintains our health. These seven doctors are 1) Dr. Sunshine or Dr. Open air, 2) Dr. Diet, 3) Dr. Quiet, 4) Dr. Smiles or Dr. Cheerfulness, 5) Dr. Cleanliness, 6) Dr. Temperance and 7) Dr. Check-up.

Prevention requires some basic knowledge about our body and how it works. If we rinse our eyes with cold water at least five times a day, probability of cataract operation is reduced by 80%. Brushing of teeth before going to sleep can save you from many teeth problems in later life.

Be Happy—Be Healthy

When you are happy, chances are that you will be healthy, and the same is true for the reverse. You will be healthy if you are happy. Health and happiness are the two sides of the same coin.

When you are happy, your energies always function better. In fact, when you are happy, you have endless energy. So just knowing a little happiness liberates you from your normal limitations of energy and capability. Our body's immune system fights more effectively when we are happy rather than depressed. When we are depressed, the number of certain disease fighting cells declines. The depressed people are more vulnerable to various illnesses. They are normally self-focused. A happy person, on the other hand, is more outgoing.

So, what exactly is happiness? It is an all-pervasive sense of well-being. Happiness is something which should outlast yesterday's moment of elation, today's buoyant mood and tomorrow's hard time.

Happiness is not necessarily linked to looks, riches or popularity. You are happy when you have a sense of psychological fullness, when you feel connected with others, when you are a person who wants to give and take, care and share. Happy people themselves have great degree of self-esteem. Optimism is another requirement to be happy-healthy. Optimist people are less bothered by failure in life.

Happiness is well within. A happy person is the one whose heart is so full of joy that nothing can add to or take away anything from him.

Remember you were on a European vacation three years back. It was a lot of fun and you were very happy. Today you are in hospital due to heart attack. Your mind is constantly under pressure. Are you happy? The answer is "no" and no one can be happy under this situation. Then, what happened to the joy and enjoyment you had three years back in Europe? The real happiness is in mind. Try to be happy by mind and healthy by body.

Be happy to be healthy and be healthy to be happy.

13

Conclusion

This is the only life we know for ever. We have no idea from where we came and where we will go after closing the eyes for the eternal journey. Nothing will last for ever on this side of the universe. Anything that comes on this planet, has to go from here. Our life span of about 80 to 100 years is nothing compared to the life on this earth which has been here for about 8 billion years. So we must enjoy every moment of life. We should try to live long with health and happiness.

By simply observing and implementing these basic but simple rules in our daily life, we can reach up to 100 years happily and healthily.

Life is like a journey by train. We board a train at a particular station and get off at a certain station. In case of a simple train journey, we know both stations but in the journey of life, we have no control over or idea about our stations. We do not know at what station we have to board the train and at what station we have to get off. The only truth we know is that we must get off the train. No one is allowed on the train of life, for ever.

100 years from now!

Just think about the situation after 100 years from now. Almost no one on this earth will be alive. The whole population will change. We do not know who will be living in our house, in our city and country. Theses occupants or residents are not yet born.

Life is the game of limited overs. Imagine since when and for how long this earth has been in existence. As per scientific calculation, its age is around eight billion years. Now compare our average life span of 80 to 100 years with this.

It is like a small black dot on a big white paper. Nobody can notice that small black dot. Whatever time we have, we should just spend it after long lasting happiness, with a cheerful mind.

Last but not Least.........

Everything discussed above is possible only if you have patience, continuation and concentration. The whole process is least expensive but its benefits are for life time.

You must have enough patience to start getting the actual benefits. Initial changes are within the body, so it will take some time to come out of body.

Every step of this process should be continual in life for a long time. If you start something today, then keep it up every day, with the exception of certain unavoidable condition or circumstances.

During the process, your concentration is required on its activities. For example, you are taking herbal juice every morning. Then think about the benefits of this herbal juice, and your body will soon get the advantages.

There are three ways to keep from getting tired and aged. "Minimize the amount you eat, meditate and do not be goal-oriented." Many people waste a lot of energy after worrying about possible outcomes and results. You can defuse the stress by living in the present moment, by refusing to wear a watch on the weekend, or by ignoring what is coming next.

We are all mortal. We will all die one day. Remember nothing lasts for ever on this side of the planet. Anything comes on this planet has to go from here. It is only a question of when and how. We have no idea from where we came and where we will go after death. What is important is that there should not be any regrets. From hugs and kisses and sorry to thank you and I love you, there should be nothing left unsaid or undone. Take time out to connect with, share a laugh, lend your shoulder and give a hug to everyone around you.

The quality of life was not determined by what happened to us, but by our own reaction to it. Though certain circumstances may be out of control, it was for us to soak up the joy and learn from the hurt. Life is not just one big high. It comes with the lows too. And what does not kill you only makes you stronger. One does not succeed at everything, but what is unacceptable is not trying.

Our past is nothing, but a collection of memories. Your future is nothing, but imagination. What you have in your control is today. Make it a happy and positive day and you will have lovely memories to look back upon. I am on this planet and I want to live, not just exist. Life is too short and wondrous to waste in grief and negativity. Live fully, live graciously and learn to be happy.

So just be happy, be merry and live the life the way it should be, because this is the only life we have on this earth and in our knowledge.

About the Author

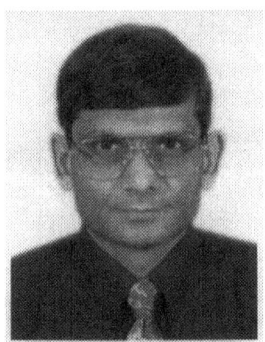

The author, Nitin M Patel, 48, is a civil engineer by profession but he has spent almost his whole life studying and analyzing Ayurveda, in India. He has devoted more than 8 years in India, after preparing this book. His personal experience and experiments are the main source of the contents of this book.

Email: nitinpatel55@hotmail.com or nitinpatel55@icenet.net

0-595-31312-4